AUTOPHAGY

EXTENDED WATER FASTING IS THE POWERFUL SECRET OF HEALING AND ANTI-AGING USING YOUR BODY'S NATURAL INTELLIGENCE

LOGAN WOLF

Healing yourself is connected with healing others.

Yoko Ono

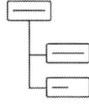

Table of Contents

DISCLAIMER

INTRODUCTION

CHAPTER 1: WHAT IS AUTOPHAGY - 1

CHAPTER 2: HOW AUTOPHAGY WORKS - 5

CHAPTER 3: THE BENEFITS OF AUTOPHAGY - 13

CHAPTER 4: HOW TO ACTIVATE AUTOPHAGY - 18

CHAPTER 5: EXTENDED WATER FASTING - 23

CHAPTER 6: INTERMITTENT FASTING - 28

CHAPTER 7: THE FASTING-MIMICKING DIET - 31

CHAPTER 8: THE BONUS WEIGHT LOSS OF AUTOPHAGY - 36

AFTERWORD - 85

MORE REFERENCES - 87

Disclaimer

This book is not intended to replace medical advice. It is not responsible for the actions and results of the reader. Please seek out the advice of a doctor before starting any health program. The author is not a medical doctor, and the information in this book is meant to supplement your health changes, not dictate them. The wonders of autophagy are still being discovered as this book was written. Please enjoy this information we provide but also be wise in consuming it.

Introduction

Congratulations on purchasing *Autophagy: Extended Water Fasting is the Powerful Secret of Healing and Anti-Aging using Your Body's Natural Intelligence* with bonus information about Intermittent Fasting and the Fasting Mimicking Diet for Weight Loss. Thank you for doing so.

The following chapters will discuss what autophagy is, why it is beneficial to your health, and why it's more than just a mere "diet fad." By reading this book, you've started on the road to cellular and bodily recovery and potentially weight loss! So, grab your preferred drink of choice, ease into your favorite chair, and let's get started.

First, let's explore what autophagy is, the man who is responsible for bringing it into the mainstream conscious, and why it won't a Nobel Prize.

Back on October 3, 2016, the Nobel Assembly at Karolinska Institute gave the Nobel Prize in Physiology or Medicine to scientist Yoshinori Ohsumi. He discovered the mechanisms of autophagy.

So, what does "autophagy" mean? The term comes from the Greek words "auto," which means "self" and "phage," which mean "eat." It sounds a bit strange, but consider it to mean "self-eating." The idea came back in the 60's around the time that researcher's first saw that our cells could kill its own innards. They did so by forming vesicles that were put into a type of recycling center, which is called the lysosome. This is where the contents were degraded. The problem with the phenomenon is that little was known about it, and therefore not much research was done regarding it. That changed, however, in the early 1990s with Doctor Yoshinori Ohsumi. He used baker's yeast to find genes that were important to the autophagy process. The yeast allowed for Ohsumi to point out the similar machinery that's used in our cells.

His discoveries created a new paradigm that helped with our understanding of cellular recycling. It opened a way to understand the importance of autophagy in our bodies, for instance, the adaptation to starvation or its response to infection. The mutations in autophagy genes could lead to disease. He also found that the autophagy process is involved in a few conditions such as cancer and neurological diseases.

The history of how we got to Ohsumi's discoveries is interesting to know. Belgian scientist Christian de Duve received the Nobel Prize in Physiology or Science 1974 for discovering the lysosome. He coined the term "autophagy" or "self-eating."

Progress was made once again in 2004 when Irwin Rose, Avram Hershko, and Aaron Ciechanover were awarded the Nobel Prize in Chemistry for discovering what is called the "ubiquitin-mediated protein degradation." They were responsible for helping us understand that proteasome degrades proteins one at a time. This opened the door to the mystery of how our cell gets rid of larger protein complexes and organelles that have been worn down. Scientists wondered if the answer was found in autophagy and what were the mechanisms that made it happen?

Scientist Yoshinori Ohsumi toiled away in his personal lab in 1988. He focused on yeast cells because they're easier to study and are a decent model of the human cells. While toiling away, he hit a significant roadblock. The problem with yeast cells is that they're small and their internal structures are not easy to tell apart when looking at them under a microscope. This made him question if autophagy even existed in them. He rethought his strategy until he found a striking revelation – the vacuoles that were chockfull of small vesicles hadn't degraded. The vesicles were autophagosomes. In layman's terms, Ohsumi had proved that autophagy existed in yeast cells! After making this significant discovery, he published his results in 1992.

Eventually, he was able to answer the question about how it worked in our own cells. Thanks to advancing technology, the research tools he needed to investigate the matter became available.

It is thanks to him and those who stepped into his big shoes that we know autophagy controls vital functions within us, including cellular components that need to be recycled and degraded. Autophagy can quickly give us fuel for energy and the elements required for renewing cellular components. This makes it very important to understanding how and why our cells respond to different types of stress such as starvation. After you've received an infection, autophagy can help you get rid of invaders like viruses and bacteria. It also contributes to the development of the embryo and cell differentiation. Autophagy can also be used in the cell to kill off damaged organelles and proteins. This, in turn, can help counteract the negative effects of aging.

His studies also helped us understand that autophagy, when disrupted, is possibly linked to Type 2 diabetes, Parkinson's diseases, and other disorders from which older people may suffer. The mutation within an autophagy gene can even bring upon genetic diseases. Research is still somewhat fresh on that matter, but it has become an essential part of the more significant conversation in the scientific realm.

In short, autophagy as a whole has a roughly fifty-year scientific history. All who contributed to the advancement of its knowledge have helped us get to where we are today and will be remembered as we advance. However, we can't ignore how important and instrumental scientist Yoshinori Ohsumi's research has been to the entire process. Without him, this book wouldn't exist!

There are other books on this subject. Thanks again for choosing this one! Every effort was made to ensure it is full of as much useful information as possible; please enjoy!

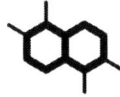

What is Autophagy?

AS WE MENTIONED in the introduction, autophagy, which is a combination of the words "self" and "eating" is known as the regulated process in which a cell in our body degrades its bad parts. The cell itself will then recycle useful chemical components for other purposes. This process then allows for autophagy to adjust the stability of protein composition within a cell in our body. This helps to prevent the building up of toxic waste products, aids in sustaining cells during periods in which our body is starving, gets rid of invading pathogens, and maintains cellular organelle function.

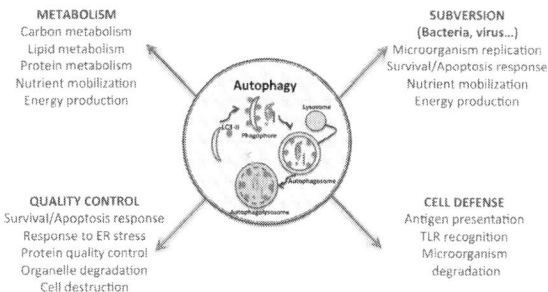

METABOLISM
Carbon metabolism
Lipid metabolism
Protein metabolism
Nutrient mobilization
Energy production

SUBVERSION
(Bacteria, virus...)
Microorganism replication
Survival/Apoptosis response
Nutrient mobilization
Energy production

QUALITY CONTROL
Survival/Apoptosis response
Response to ER stress
Protein quality control
Organelle degradation
Cell destruction

CELL DEFENSE
Antigen presentation
TLR recognition
Microorganism
degradation

Consider autophagy to be when your body creates a dumpster, also known as your autophagosome. What it does is collect cellular components and takes them to the local cellular "recycling center" which is scientifically known as the lysosome. This is where it gets broken down into small parts which are then repurposed into new pieces of machinery. New cells.

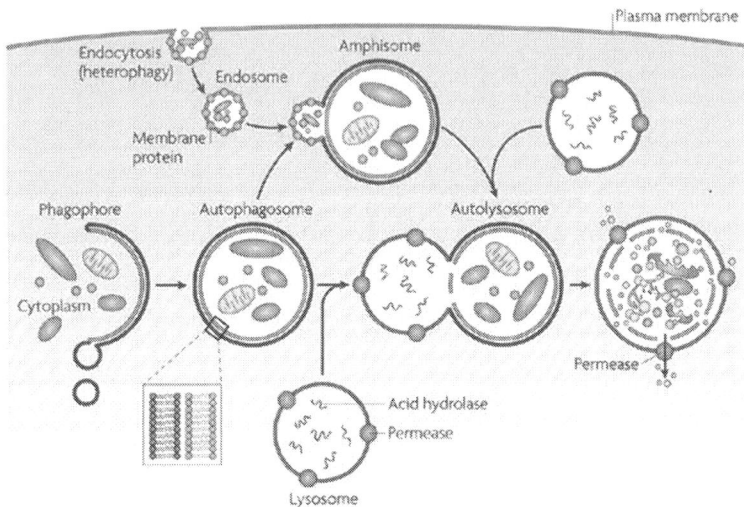

AUTOPHAGY: DEFINITIONS

A process that is very similar to it is called apoptosis, which is also known as "programmed cell death." After a set amount of time dividing, the cells are programmed to perish. This process may sound disturbing at first, but it is actually crucial in keeping a healthy body. For instance, consider it like having a vehicle. You buy it, you grow to adore it, and you create memories with it. It's is a part of your life, and you take it places. However, as the years go by, your car naturally suffers wear and tear. After a while, as much as you love it, you have to let it go because it's eventually going to take a lot of money to keep it going. Moreover, even with the maintenance, your car breaks down continuously. You'll have to finally get another one because it's eventually leading to the junkyard. You don't want to keep it around by the time it becomes something that'll sit in your backyard, so you end up getting rid of it. You then got out and purchase a new one.

This analogy helps us to understand what's going on in our bodies. Our cells slowly become useless and old. It is ideal for them to be programmed to die when they no longer can do what they were built to do in the first place. This is what science calls "apoptosis." Cells are destined to die before they're even born, that is, after they've exhausted their usefulness. Taking it back to our car analogy, after a certain time has past and our car is no longer able to work, and then we get a new one. The good news with this process though is that you don't have to worry about having to "purchase" anything. With autophagy, your body will do it on its own.

When our bodies are running well, and the cells are running smoothly, autophagy happens at a lower level, which helps us recycle these worn-down cellular mechanisms. We're in a good maintenance mode. Things can become complicated when they're stressed, however. In the cellular scenario, stress comes from when our bodies don't have enough nutrients or energy, from un-recycled and dysfunctional components, or when microbes invade them. Autophagy then gets "turned up" because it's going to work to help save us. Science calls this the "stress mode."

This process also happens on what science calls the sub-cellular level. Returning to the car analogy, you don't really have to get rid of the entire car, per se. At the time, all you need to do is replace a part, like putting in a new battery. Out with the old and in with the new! Killing off the entire cell is what makes apoptosis different from autophagy. For the process of autophagy, the sub-cellular organelles are killed off, and new ones are rebuilt to take over for the old ones. Organelles, old cell membranes, and other parts of a cell that are cast-off are able to be removed. This happens by transferring it to the lysosome which is an organelle that contains enzymes that help to degrade proteins.

One thing that makes autophagy so remarkable is the process is in which it occurs happens when there is what science calls cellular stress. That is if the cells lack specific nutrients, or they're deprived of energy, or become damaged for some reason, the "stress response" is activated and autophagy happens in a higher speed. This causes cell function to improve when we, and thus our bodies, are under duress. We'll explore more of this phenomenon in chapters two and four.

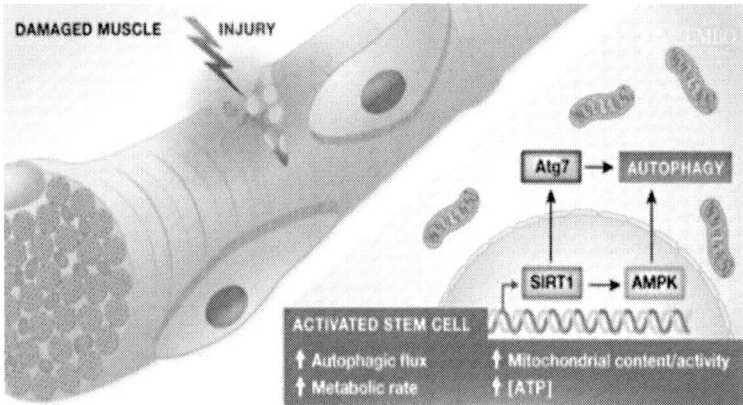

Ultimately, the science revolving around autophagy tells us is that it helps to make our bodies work better. By clearing out all of the cellular "junk" within us, we are then clearing a way for cells to recreate themselves with new components. This biological upgrade can be seen as giving our car a new engine. It helps to keep us "running."

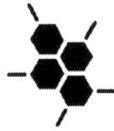

How Autophagy Works

BEFORE THE "HOW," there was the discovery, and that was in the middle of the 1950s as Sam Clark Jr. from the School of Medicine at Washington University in St. Louis took a gander through his electron microscope at these newly born mouse kidneys and noticed something that he didn't see there the other times he looked through the microscope. As reported, he describes it as the appearance of a membrane-bound structure found within the cytoplasm of the new kidney cells. What was interesting was the structures seemed to have changed mitochondria.

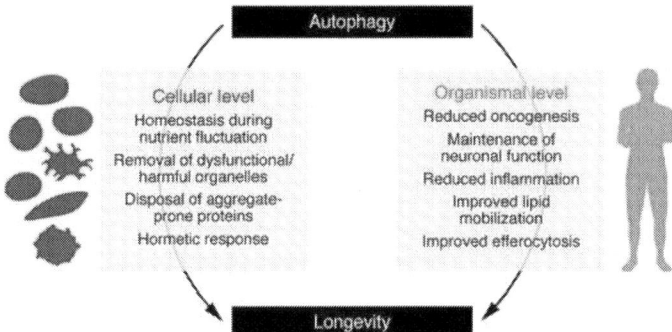

Autophagy

Cellular level
Homeostasis during nutrient fluctuation
Removal of dysfunctional/ harmful organelles
Disposal of aggregate-prone proteins
Hormetic response

Organismal level
Reduced oncogenesis
Maintenance of neuronal function
Reduced inflammation
Improved lipid mobilization
Improved efferocytosis

Longevity

Afterward, Clark published his new findings, and a few independent researchers supported his conclusions. The likes of which included Alex Novikoff from the Albert Einstein College of Medicine. He used the word cytolyses for the structures. He and his colleague Edward Essner wrote in their research that "within these cytolyses remarkable events are in progress," and that the "cytoplasm has somehow found its way inside the droplets and is apparently in the process of digestion."

Those were the first research-oriented footsteps for what we do not call autophagy.

What defines autophagy is what is known as the formation of the transient double-membrane structure which is called a phagophore. This differentiates from the secretory transport vesicles, as they happen to pull away from an organelle with stuff already within it. The phagophore gets its stuff during its initial assemblage. The structure might create de novo within the cytoplasm, which will become what science calls a free-standing structure. It may also come in contact with an organelle like that of the endoplasmic reticulum. The phagophore then expands which gives it great flexibility to carry even more stuff within it. As it continues to swell, it impounds the cytoplasmic parts, which include lipids, proteins, and possibly the whole organelle. Once this load is held, the phagophore closes up and then ages into an autophagosome, with the held load now enveloped within the lumen of this partition. The autophagosome then delivers the load by the membrane fusion into the lytic compartments (which are lysosomes within metazoans and vacuoles in plants and fungi) for them to be degraded and recycled. And it was with this scientifically complex process that caught the attention of Novikoff and Clark those many years ago, which led to what we now know as autophagy!

Autophagy itself can be broken down into two bigger categories

– the selective and the nonselective. Each of them is based on what is being eaten. Currently, research knows more about macroautophagy. This contains the delivery of cellular components sent to the lysosome, which is known as the vacuole within plants and fungi. This happens by a double-membrane bound structure. There are also two other forms, which are chaperone-mediated autophagy and microautophagy. The lysosome encloses on and confiscates nearby cellular materials which are ready to be destroyed and recycled. The chaperone-mediated autophagy, on the other hand, is a particular protein-deterioration process that relies on dedicated transporters of lysosomes.

Nowadays, autophagy is considered an essential process for maintaining an excellent cellular balance in our bodies. It is also crucial for reacting to body stressors, like when the body is nutrient-deprived, which can compromise cellular survival. The cell is bare to these stresses and the autophagy, which is usually at a lower level, is then kicked up to deal with the heightened stress. It increases requisitioning and mortification of parts of the cell, which releases macromolecules back into the cytosol. They then powerup the critical metabolic reactions and thus create vital energy.

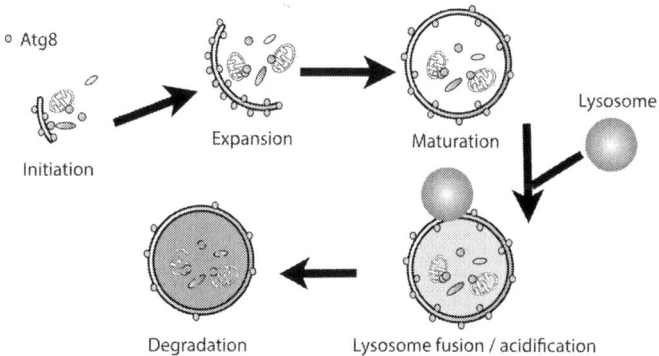

Atg8

Initiation

Expansion

Maturation

Lysosome

Lysosome fusion / acidification

Degradation

The fact that autophagy contributes to the cellular health of our bodies under both stress and normal conditions shows us just how important it is to regulate our cells. Autophagy has become instrumental in understanding the development of mammals. More recent research has shown us that autophagy is an essential modulator of a vast array of disorders and diseases. Understanding the involvement of autophagy within our bodies helps explain the way in which we get (and can prevent) diseases. While we know the key points of autophagy, there is still a long way to go.

There are a few catabolic paths within a cell that can break down the larger molecules in our body. One that is pretty notorious is the conjugation of a smaller protein which is called a "ubiquitin." The process takes this to another cellular protein which is then followed by successive addition of the ubiquitin molecules which generate a polyubiquitin chain. This can tap that protein for destruction via the proteasome thus giving us amino acids. These mechanisms of deterioration are found in other biological polymers like lipids and carbohydrates.

Autophagy is unique in that is has flexibility of autophagosome cargo selection and size. It can push for the destruction of a large group and variety of substrates, which helps to enable cells to quickly and effectively create recycled essential "building blocks" needed for a wide range of deficiencies in the nutritional realm. Autophagy also is the only passageway that can degrade a full organelle. It can do so in both a targeted and essential process in which the body must be put back in cellular homeostasis.

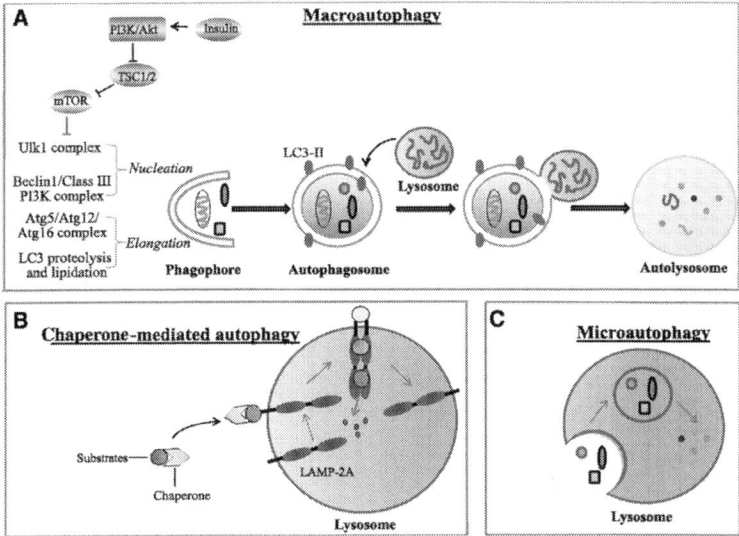

The body regulates autophagy to make sure that it kicks into high gear only when it's required and that it happens in a timely manner. The central metabolic sensor of our cell, which as the TOR complex 1, is responsive to how much amino acid is available to the body. The TOR complex 1, also known as TORC1, is inactive when the cells are starving of those molecules. This then allows for the promotion of the increase of autophagy. In the meantime, molecular regulators keep an eye out for cells and watch out for the number of different nutrients, such as ATP energy, or glucose, and will activate autophagy when these nutrients hit a critical low. Once this process starts, several ATG proteins come together, like a superhero squad and coordinate the creation of the phagophore and initiate the steps for autophagy. The Yeast ATG genes, as we've discussed earlier were discovered in the 90s, which helped to transcend autophagy research. The experiments that used the budding yeast was a significant step forward to help scientists understand the basics of autophagy. It was during this time in which the research transcended into or organisms which then made it easier for scientists to see how it works in the human body. It showed us that it was an evolutionary part of our survival!

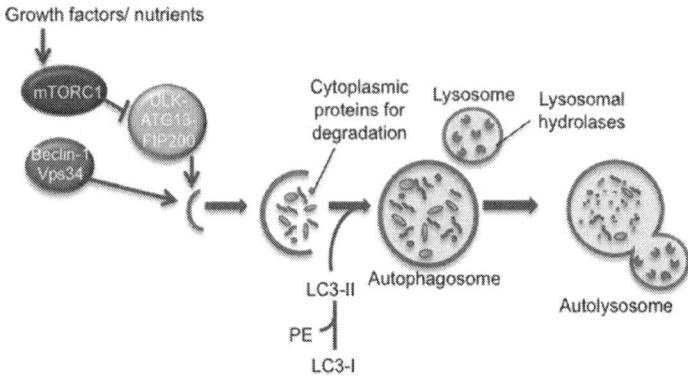

In a more general term, autophagy works in a "survival of the fittest" type of regime. Our cells are born to consume weak parts of themselves. Doing this makes it much stronger. Consider it like the Darwinian concept literally on a molecular level. The parts that are stronger will eat those that are weak. It's a natural process that keeps the body functioning. Just as we are evolving, so are our bodies' cells. They're becoming capable of consuming functional materials which have no more value to them in their current state.

Let us take a more in-depth look at the Chaperone-mediated autophagy that we mentioned earlier. Also known as CMA for short, it is about the chaperone-dependent assortment of soluble cytosolic proteins. They are sought out by lysosomes and sent across the lysosome membrane for decomposition. The unique features of this category of autophagy are the discrimination of the proteins destroyed in this path and the movement of these proteins across the lysosomal membrane. It happens without the requirement of added vesicles.

Now, let's take a look at microautophagy.

Unlike Chaperone-mediated autophagy and Macroautophagy, microautophagy is a type of autophagic path that is referred by direct lysosome coverage within the cytoplasmic items. The cytoplasmic material is collected into the lysosome within an unpredictable process of membrane enclosing and unfolding into itself. Microautophagy path is particularly essential for cells to survive through the process of starvation. Microautophagy is considered a non-selective route, but there are several different events of selective microautophagy-oriented paths that are initiated when certain conditions are met. These three are Micromitophagy, Piecemeal microautophagy of the nucleus, and macropexophagy.

When combined, microautophagy and macroautophagy are important because of their nutrient recycling abilities when the body is in starvation mode. Microautophagy comes with the degradation of the lipids that assimilate into vesicles, which adjusts the arrangement of the lysosomal. The microautophagy path acts as one of the tools of glycogen delivery within the lysosomes. This autophagic pathway submerges multivesicular bodies molded after endocytosis. Because of this, it plays a vital role in the turnover of membrane proteins. Additionally, microautophagy is linked to organellar size upkeep, the modification from starvation-created progression arrest to logarithmic development, cell survival through nitrogen deprivation, and confirmation of biological membranes.

Lipophagy is another form of autophagy. This type of autophagy comes with the degradation of lipids. It's a function that's existed within both us human and fungus-based cells. The role that it plays within plants, however, is still relatively unknown to us. When lipophagy happens, it targets the lipid structures in our bodies with are called LDs, or lipid droplets. They're organelles that have a core mostly made of TAGs or triacylglycerols. They contain a layer of phospholipids and membrane proteins. The main lipophagic pathway, within our cells, is through the engulfment of lipid droplets by the phagosphere. We first learned of lipophagy when scientists discovered it within mice, and the findings were released in 2009.

We're also still learning about Mitophagy, which is the selective deterioration of mitochondria via autophagy. It happens mostly to defective mitochondria after stress or damage. Mitophagy helps to turnover mitochondria and helps prevent the adding up of dysfunctional mitochondria. This keeps cellular degeneration at bay! The process is facilitated by Atg32 (found in yeast), NIX and its "supervisor" known as BNIP3. PINK1 and parkin proteins control the process of Mitophagy. The circumstance of mitophagy happens to both damaged and undamaged mitochondria.

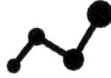

3

The Benefits of Autophagy

AFTER A RELATIVELY DAUNTING scientific explanation about what autophagy is and the different types of autophagy that exist, let's take a break and look at what the actual benefits are to activating it.

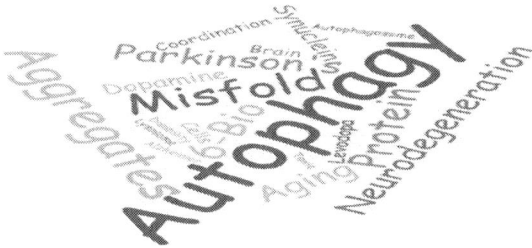

1. It helps in the fight against cancer.

Autophagy helps us to survive when our body is in starvation mode. Scientific research tells us that cancer was one of the primary diseases associated with autophagy; however, the way in which it works with cancer cells and the role autophagy has in them is still mostly unknown. At the earlier stages of cancer, autophagy usually acts as a tumor suppressor, which allows the cells to get rid of damaged cellular parts and decrease DNA and ROS damage. In the advanced stages of the development of a tumor, it could help cancer cells survive under low-oxygen and low-nutrient situations.

Autophagy, most importantly, plays a role in how cancer responds to therapy. The reason being is that most cancer therapies create damage and stress to the cells to kill them. This makes treatment that uses autophagy a potentially good or potentially bad solution. It also depends on the type of cancer. We also have to consider what stage the disease is in and what type of autophagy and the duration of it. A few studies have revealed that increased autophagy leads to the resistance of both chemotherapy and radiotherapy, but a few others revealed that a slew of anticancer drugs helps to stimulate autophagy-oriented cell death within cancer cells.

Autophagy is clearly becoming a place of interest to clinical research as some of the more recently approved anti-cancer stratagems noted as inducing autophagy. Learning more about this can help with creating medications and radiation treatments that can aid in getting rid of tumors.

We have to be careful when looking at the way autophagy affects someone with cancer because there have been some research results which tell us that it can go into various, somewhat unpredictable manners. This makes autophagy quite the mysterious entity, but we can't ignore that it has had some promising results.

Autophagy has been linked with cancer and other illnesses such as Parkinson's disease. Currently, medical processes using the recent discoveries of Ohsumi are now happening around the world. The vital role that it plays in chemotherapeutic drugs and radiation is growing. Research shows that there are four different functional forms of autophagy which can happen when the body is responding to chemotherapy or radiation. They are: cytostatic, cytotoxic, non-protective, and cytoprotective. None of them have a specified result that scientists can predict yet. The line between protecting cancer and tumor cells and autophagy deleting them are still quite blurred. Some scientists suggest that this is where next to put research focus.

2. It can improve your cognition and the health of
your brain

Neurologists will say to you that there are a set of metabolic processes that are important to your body to help keep its health. This is important to the brain as well. Inducing autophagy onto your body can help to stimulate the brain. The way it works is that by fasting, you're increasing the circulating levels of a few neurotrophic components. They're biomolecules which support the differentiation, survival, and growth of neurons. The endgame of this is a more enhanced network elasticity which is essential for our ability to learn new things. It also helps us to become more resilient to stress and increases our mitochondria, which helps to raise cognitive energy.

Inducing autophagy, or fasting can also help to reduce oxidative stress in the brain by both stimulating the elimination of broken molecules and arousing the creation of endogenous antioxidants. Overall, this means that autophagy can help impact your brain's performance. The science behind autophagy and illnesses is still somewhat new, but some research shows that it can help to reduce the neuronal dysfunction that comes with diseases like Parkinson's and Alzheimer's.

3. It can help reverse and slow down aging markers.

Aging, from the scientific perspective, can be defined as the slow but overtime noticeable accretion of organelles and proteins in our cells. This can lead to the eventual death or dysfunction of cells. Consider autophagy to be an aging reversal, as helps to give your body a cellular jumpstart. It stimulates your cells to get rid of parts of cells that are no longer needed and helps your body continue to create new cells. These cells are critical because they are the ones that help stave off things like cancer.

4. It can help improve your body's composition.

We live in a world where calorie intake is what we're told to look at almost exclusively when it comes to dieting, eating right, and watching the health of bodies; however, that's not always the case. While calories are necessary, we can't forget that body composition is based on our hormonal state.

Inducing autophagy can help increase our adiponectin levels and increase our sensitivity to insulin. Both of these are critical hormonal factors, and determine if the fat that already exists within us gets oxidized, meaning used for energy and if future caloric intake gets stored as fat or used by the body immediately. These hormonal changes are excellent, and persist after your fasting period is complete. While you will more than likely run a calorie deficit during your fasting days, the hormonal changes will have much more impact on your body's composition over the weeks and months. Yay for fasting and longevity.

One of the big myths that gym-going types have is that fasting will break down muscles for energy. There is some truth to this under dire conditions, but it's also easy to avoid if you're smart about your fasting cycle. If you do it right, short-term fasting can help increase lipolysis which is fat burning, and you can ideally maintain your muscle growth.

5. It can help improve your digestion

Instinctively, inducing autophagy is like a type of rest on your digestive system. It allows the gastrointestinal tract, also known as GI for short, to relax for a while. Ideally, this helps to produce both reduced intestinal inflammation and to help improve the contraction of the GI muscles indigestion. Collectively, they help to enhance the absorption of nutrients and aid in the quality of your bowel movements. While the research is still pretty fresh, there are hints that autophagy may help stimulate the growth of a different species of bacteria in our guts which can improve the fat burning process! This is pretty exciting!

6. It can help your cardiovascular health

Inducing autophagy can help to reduce your heart rate and blood pressure all the while raising the parasympathetic tone, which is a crucial gauge for the health of our cardiovascular systems. In the most generic terms, the strength of our cardiovascular system to forms of stress improves after inducting autophagy.

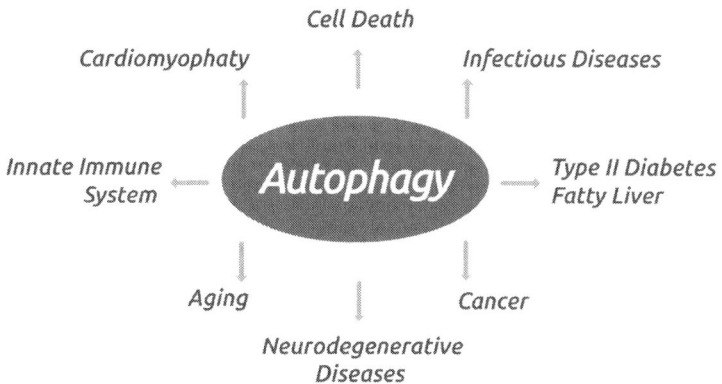

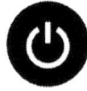

4

How to Activate Autophagy

SO, the big question is: when does autophagy happen? Well, it is activated in all the cells but increases when we're in a stressful situation, such as being nutrient deprived because of fasting or starvation. The way we activate this is to put our body in the process of dealing with "good stresses." Two methods of doing this are exercising, and temporarily restricting our calorie intake. As we've mentioned the previous chapter, these are linked with beneficial factors in controlling weight, the longevity of our lives, and inhibiting the destruction of cells which protects against age-related diseases. Here's an extended breakdown of how we can activate autophagy.

1. Fasting.

When looking into dieting and lifestyle changes that you can learn to control, one of the things you will want to consider doing when inducing autophagy is fasting. It is one of the most effective ways of inducing autophagy. The concept of fasting is quite simple – you don't eat for a certain amount of time, though you are allowed to drink water and occasionally other liquids such as tea and coffee.

One way many people have recently started fasting is through what is called "Intermittent fasting." This is a type of fasting that encompasses time-restricted eating. IMF, as it's known for short, can be done in different forms, which will discuss later in this book. Mainly, this branched out the type of fasting that called Alternate Day fasting, which limits your daily eating window to between 4-8 hours per day and then fasting for the remainder of the day.

One of the big questions you might have right now is how long does one have to fast to initiate autophagy. Some studies have suggested that we should fast between twenty-four to forty-eight hours to have the strongest effect on our bodies. The problem with this is that is doesn't always work for everyone. It would be better to start closer to twelve to thirty-six hours at a time.

An ideal way to start is to eat just one or two meals a day instead of eating smaller meals and snacks throughout the day. If you are usually finishing up your day and having your last meal around six or seven in the evening, consider trying to fast until around seven the next morning. In more intense fasting scenarios, you can consider fasting until eleven in the morning or even twelve in the afternoon.

You can also consider occasionally doing a two to three days fast, and extend it even longer once you've adapted to fasting. If you're following the alternate day fasting, then you will be restricting your calorie intake to around 500 but then taking in enough calories that feel satiating when you're on your non-fasting days.

2. Take the Ketogenic Diet into consideration.

The ketogenic (or keto) diet is a high-fat, low carbohydrate diet that works well with fasting. Called KD for short, it involves having about seventy-five percent or more of your daily calories coming from fat, and less than five to ten percent of your calories coming from carbs. This diet thus forces your body to take on some more significant changes because your metabolic pathways shift so that your begin utilizing your body's fat for fuel instead of the glucose from carbohydrates.

Some of the foods you'll want to consider if your going the KD route is high-fat, whole foods. Consider stuff like nuts, seeds, avocado, fermented cheeses, meat products from grass-fed animals, ghee, butter from grass-fed animals, eggs, olive oil, and coconut oil. The response from your body is fascinating. It will begin to produce ketone bodies that have protective factors in them. Some research implies that ketosis can help induce starvation-style autophagy, which also has neuroprotective functions to it. It should be noted that these are mainly from animal research, so the conclusions from these studies are far off.

3. Exercising

As we mentioned earlier, exercising is a good stress that can induce autophagy. Recent research findings have told us that exercise helps to induce autophagy within multiple organs which are involved in metabolic regulation, like adipose and pancreas tissue, and liver and muscle tissue. The reason why exercise is considered a form of stress is that it breaks down tissues which cause them to be repaired and come back stronger once they've grown. We currently don't know the specific amount of exercise you need to do to induce autophagy, but research implies that the more intense workouts are most beneficial.

For cardiac and skeletal muscle tissue, some experts suggest as little as 30 minutes of exercising can be enough to induce autophagy. The bigger question, however, is if you can exercise while fasting. This is largely based on the individual. Some people can. Some people find that they're more energetic once they adapt to fasting, which gives them the motivation to exercise.

4. Going on a protein fast.

One fast you may want to consider if the protein fast. What you do in this fast is one or twice a week, your limit how much protein you eat by about fifteen to twenty-five grams a day. This will give you a body a full day to recycle the proteins, which can help decrease inflammation and clean your cells without the fear of muscle loss. Autophagy is triggered when the body has no choice but to feast on its own toxins and protein.

5. Performing High-Intensity Interval Training (HIIT for short).

HIIT is an excellent way to bring on autophagy. High-intensity exercise puts you in a state of "good" stress because it stresses your body out enough that you provoke a biochemical change. Your body will have just enough impact loads to make your muscles sturdier, but not enough that it will do you any harm. Some research says that you should consider approximately twenty to thirty minutes a day to give your longevity an optimal boost.

In this "less is more" type of exercise for encouraging autophagy, you'll want to consider resistance training and weightlifting exercises for about 30 minutes every other day. This is ideal for activating autophagy. The goal here is to get short-term critical stress because autophagy does well with creating stress in intervals.

6. Don't underestimate the power of restorative sleeping.

Don't forget that autophagy still happens while you're asleep as well. Take into consideration the way you sleep. There are some periods-of-sleep quizzes out there that can help you identify what type of sleep personality you have. Your sleep personality takes into account how long you sleep and in what cycles. It is crucial because understanding your sleep cycle can either enhance or ruin your day. This can help set your body up to activate autophagy through your sleep and wake cycles.

5

Extended Water Fasting

FASTING IS HARD. Fasting for two weeks or more is even harder. So why would you do it? Only a small percentage of people within the western hemisphere take on water fasting, and an even lower percentage of people who do so will do it for fourteen days or more. The bigger question is why? For some people there really isn't a need. For the cleansing and healing of the body in our daily lives, the occasional seven to ten days fast, in combination with a regular series of shorter fasts like the thirty-six-hour water fast will keep you in excellent condition.

That being said, if you want to reach the deepest sector of healing through fasting you'll want to condition yourself to do a longer fast. For example, particular physical illnesses demand more time cleansing and are considered incurable by most modern medicine. While you should first always consult a doctor, such diseases as autoimmune disorders, tumors, chronic high blood pressure, multiple sclerosis, and Type-2 diabetes can be treated using extended water fasting.

Likewise, going on an extended water fast can help you cleanse yourself profoundly both physically and mentally. Fasting on this level sounds almost mythical and brings to mind some figures from western civilization's past such as the biblical Moses and the Greek Pythagoras. They both went on a cleanse for forty days, which depending on how you interpret it will either literally mean forty days, or for an extended amount of time. Some people consider that the average body stores about 100,000 calories within it, and the best way to tap into that energy source would be to teach your body what is there. Then your body will eat what it has stored instead of anticipating, and waiting for your next meal.

In one aspect of extended water fasting, those following it have come to deem it "extended healing fast," because of how the process works. For the sake of understanding this more, let's describe more in the manner of eastern over western medical terms. Consider this: your body, during the first seven to ten days of the fast, is going through what is called a "healing crisis." This healing crisis is when the symptoms of older illnesses, injuries, and traumas stored within your body begin to reemerge. The good news: this is also the time that your body starts to expel them. This early process is similar to what happens when you extend the fast further, aiming for around fourteen days. By doing so, you're tapping into even deeper old illnesses and damage in your body, which means that you're going for an even deeper cleanse. This second healing crisis is for deeper issues embedded in the body. You go from cleansing the daily toxins from your body to tapping into things that were there for years!

Some fasters recommend that for the deepest cleanse and for those who are trying to expel serious health issues from their bodies, in both the physical and spiritual manner, you will want to consider going even farther and longer into the cleanse. Some people who've been doing for a while have gone for twenty, thirty, even the biblical forty days of extended water fasting. You're tapping into more profound "healing crises" when you do this, but the time it takes becomes vaguer.

Not everyone hits an intense "healing crisis" when doing the extended fasting. In some cases, the symptoms of certain illnesses or personal traumas are too diverse. In these scenarios, when there is not a clear indication of what your body is working on, it can make it hard to determine for how long you should fast. This is another reason why you should always, *always* do extended fasting under the supervision of a medical expert. They will keep you from overstepping your body's nutritional competences because, as awesome as extended fasting sounds, you are still pushing your body past its previous physical limits.

If you do happen to move forward with your fasting, there will undoubtedly come the point at which you are turning the fasting process into actual starvation. You don't want to get to this point! Remember that once your body had depleted its storage of fats; it will start feasting on your muscle tissue and on your internal organs. This will have the opposite effect on you as you start to damage our body. This is when you'll get into extreme hunger. You'll notice that your body will start cramping up because after you've exhausted your body's fat through ketosis, you'll eventually begin to want another form of fuel which comes from the glucose. The Problem is that your body will begin to extract is from your muscles, thus leaving you with depleted electrolytes, which are your body's blood salts. This is the reason for why you'd want to have your doctor test your blood while you are fasting as well, especially if you have a history of blood pressure issues.

If your body feels comfortable with the 3-day water fast and can make the shift into ketosis without issue, then perhaps it's time that you look into doing the seven to ten-day water fast. The reason being is that it's at this point that you truly being to draw on the energy from your fat cells which the process of detoxification truly starts to hit the higher gears.

The process may seem harder in the first three days, versus the extended fast and that's because your body is working its hardest during the first three days while it's starting the ketosis cycle. This is the time in which your body's "fuel tank" is "running on empty." The good news is that from day three on, ketosis (and autophagy) continues to become more active, and therefore you'll start feeling fuller of energy and lighter. At this point, your body may feel like it's in celebratory mode as it doesn't feel the pressure to consume on a daily basis. The elation of the moment may even make you want to stop eating in general – But that's definitely NOT what you want to do, especially since the feeling will not last. Fasting doesn't mean that you stop eating. You're human. Your body needs food, eventually.

Your metabolism begins to establish itself by the end of the first day, and your digestive system finally shuts down its normal function. The consequence is that many of your hunger pains tend to quiet down during this period. You'll want to consider what you'll eat in the transition period both after and before a fast that lasts longer than three days. This is important because the last thing you want is for your body to the digestive system to shut down while there is food still within your body. The food that is doesn't process will sit inside you and thus begin to rot and therefore leave you more toxins, which completely counters the whole reason for the fasting process. Consider your digestive system to be like a bear that's in hibernation after the third day. You can't just shove it awake and expect it to function like it never went into hibernation. It takes time for it to start up again, so you'll want to eat smaller, easily digestible proportions of foods. That last thing you'll want to do is go from not eating and then head to the nearest McDonald's and get a big burger meal. It'll sit in your stomach feel like you swallowed a giant rock. On top of this, the digestive process will take forever because it's only recently waking up.

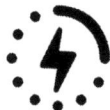

6

Intermittent Fasting

STARVATION AND FASTING ARE two different entities. Starvation is complete deprivation and fasting is taking control of your body's regulation of food. Fasting is done voluntarily and is used to create a healthier body and spirit, among other things. Food is readily available to you, but you're basically choosing not to eat. This can be beneficial to you and done in any period of time. It can happen from just a few hours to days and even weeks. You can begin a fast at any time, and you can also end it at will. Once again, it's all about control. Your reasoning can be just as varied too.

There are some standard durations for how long some people will fast, which mostly depends on which type of fast you're doing. Fasting, in general, doesn't have a set duration. You can fast between dinner and the next day's breakfast, which is roughly twelve to fourteen hours. This leads us to a discussion about intermittent fasting.

Intermittent fasting first and foremost isn't a diet. It focuses more on the pattern of your eating habits. It is a way to schedule your meals so that you get the most benefit out of them. In other words, this form of fasting isn't changing what you eat, but changes when you eat.

One of the things that make this fasting process beneficial is because it's an excellent way to get lean without going on one of the crazier diets we see popping up every year. In most cases, you'll be trying to keep your calories the same as you start this process of fasting. Many people will eat bigger meals during a short frame of time. It's also an excellent way to keep muscle mass while trying to get leaner!

The main thing that many people want when trying this particular fasting process is to lose body fat. Intermittent fasting has become of the most straightforward strategies for getting rid of bad weight off our bodies, all while keeping the good weight. Dieting, being healthier, and such are all significant lifestyle changes and can feel like huge mountains that people will be too scared to climb. Luckily intermittent dieting makes it so that it's actually pretty easy because the changes you're making don't feel like night and day.

To understand how intermittent fasting works, let's first look at two states in which your body lives – the fed state and the fasting state. When your body is in the fed state, you're eating, and your body is digesting and absorbing that food. In most cases, the cycle begins when you begin eating and lasts for roughly three to five hours because you're digesting and absorbing the food. Your body has a hard time burning fat in this state. Your insulin levels are high in this state, and that prevents fat-burning.

After a set amount of time, your body will go into a post-absorption state in which it will no longer be processing your food. This state can last from eight to twelve hours after your last meal, and that is when you hit your fasting state. It is easier for your body to burn fat when you in this state because the insulin levels of it are low. Your body can begin to burn fat that's been inaccessible during the fed state. It's rare that our bodies stay in the fat burning state because we don't enter the fasting state until 12 hours after our last meal. This is why many people have started intermittent fasting, and this is why many people who did don't change their eating habits.

To start intermittent dieting, you may want to start as early as when you wake up. Instead of eating breakfast, you'll have a glass of water and then start your day. The beauty of this form of intermittent fasting is that there is less for you to cook because you're eating one less meal a day.

Intermittent fasting helps with restricting calories, which some scientists have said can help prolong your life. You're teaching your body, in a way, to survive more because it's put in a stressful situation when you're fasting. Intermittent fasting helps to activate the mechanisms for extending life through calorie restriction.

Intermittent fasting is similar to dieting because it is easy to understand. However, unlike dieting, isn't hard to execute. The difficulties come from more of the contemplation about doing it then the actual doing it. For intermittent fasting, you're basically going without food for a specific portion of the day. You can skip breakfast, and for some, even lunch, and then you'll be able to eat dinner.

7

▶II

The Fasting-Mimicking Diet

THE FASTING-MIMICKING DIET is one that can boast of being both scientific and nutrient-dense, and science is even telling us that there may be a significant advantage for your long-term health. What makes mimicking different is that it isn't a full-on fasting process. It's a good alternative for those who aren't ready to jump into the deeper end of fasting. To better understand what the fasting-mimicking diet is all about, let's go over the general information in this chapter.

At its core, fasting-mimicking is a modified form of fasting. It differs itself from a traditional fast because you're not entirely abstaining yourself from food. You still eat, but what you eat and how much you eat is changed, and this is what produces some therapeutic benefits of fasting without the stress and anxiety that comes with initial fasting. This diet tends to last for around five days, and it follows a careful protocol that's low in protein, carbs, and calories, but is also high in fat. Your calorie intake is set to around forty percent of your usual consumption. This will allow for your body to stay nourished to an adequate level, which diminishes the stress of normal fasting because you're still getting nutrients and electrolytes. You get the best of both methods as you can fast without the initial stress but still reap the benefits. The problem is that not everyone's body can handle the water-fasting approach. This is where Dr. Longo's research comes in.

They created the fasting-mimicking diet. The benefits have shown that it can reduce cancer incidence, protect your body from the loss of bone density, promote neurogenesis, protect the body from chemotoxicity, stimulate our stem cell production, regenerate what is known as our "beta cells," which are linked with Type 1 and Type 2 Diabetes, remyelinate neuron sheaths which are related to multiple sclerosis, and prolong your life. It's worth noting that these tests have yet to be done on humans within a wider span; however, there was a large clinical trial that helped with some healthy adults. It showed that three cycles of the diet were able to lower the markers of chronic diseases, lower cholesterol, lower blood pressure, and lower levels of c-reactive protein which is a marker of inflammation, all while preserving lean body mass.

Dr. Valter Longo created the diet, and the research behind it is quite fascinating. For more than twenty years, Dr. Longo and his team studied what science calls "nutrient sensing pathways" within our cells. Much like the research revolving around autophagy, Dr. Longo's work is also linked with aging, cancer, and neurological diseases associated with age. The results from the science showed that there were benefits to fasting such as living longer due to cell destruction and regeneration and even helping to prevent terminal illnesses.

If not done correctly, long-term fasting and calorie restriction can be harmful to your body. This is why fasting-mimicking is so innovative. It's more effective and safer in this aspect.

It differs from traditional fasting in that the risk of having your body eat the muscle away after it reaches a certain level of starvation goes away. You don't run the risk of killing your metabolism. It basically "tricks" your body because you're reducing the caloric intake just enough to feel like you're fasting, so it activates autophagy and you get most of the benefits of traditional fasting.

A chunk of research has shown us that the best results during the fasting-mimicking process will show after five days or when your glucose ketone index falls below 1.0. You need not worry though, as even if you do it for three to seven days, you will still have beneficial results. You're meant to repeat the process about twice a year, and some people have even done it as frequently as once a month. This is where asking a professional for help will come in handy. Each of our bodies is different, and your normal is going to be different someone else's normal.

One thing you may want to do is measure certain biomarkers. This is a good way to keep track of your fasting outcomes. It will also keep you on track in general if you're a visual person and need a certain amount of structure to succeed. You can do so by getting lab tests done before and after the fast alongside measuring your blood glucose and ketones daily and checking on your weight fluctuations.

One thing you may also want to do is set up your environment to help prepare for the fast. This can be a simple as informing family and friends that you'll come in contact with during this period what you're up to and why it is important for them to support you. Moreover, the small yet helpful thing to do would be to get rid of any snack foods within your home and working area. The temptation may not seem like it'll be there at first, but trust me, once you're in the middle of the fasting process, that Snicker's bar that you kept in your drawer will seem like a golden pass to heaven. So why risk it? Also, be sure to give yourself time. We live busy lives, and your body will be going through quite a bit with the fasting process. You're going to feel tired at times so make sure to give yourself time to sleep. Sleep, besides water, is the second most important part of this process. Be sure to give yourself some time to exercise but do so at a lighter pace. You'll get to a point where you'll be able to, but at the beginning, go easy on yourself. Baby steps!

The fasting-mimicking diet is a five-day, plant-based meal plan. It continually gets mixed up with the Ketogenic Diet, but it is unique. The diet comes within a box. The box contains everything you'll need for you five days of fasting. What you get are an energy drink, algae oil, olives, kale crackers, tea, nut bars, and soups. The diet itself contains a measured amount of calorie intakes that starts with 1,110 for the first day and leans down to 800-700 during the proceeding days.

For those who are interested in starting the diet and getting a box, you can do so by going to the main site for Prolon at Prolon-FMD.com.

Some people have decided to go on their own as far as doing the fasting, meaning they didn't go the Prolon route. Some people who are starting the fasting say that it's easier to get into the fast by eating slightly higher calories on the first day of the fast. Many estimate around fifty percent of their total intake. They then reduce it to about thirty-five to forty percent of the sum of the entire caloric intake. If you try this, you'll want to stick with the percentages. Also, consider how and when you'll be eating during the day. You'll also want to consume stuff that is easily digestible, and you'll want to make sure to eat it in smaller amounts. Your stomach will thank you!

The good news is that for you coffee and tea drinkers, a cup of tea or black coffee a day is typically allowed, but it's not necessary for those who may not want to drink them. The thing you'll have to make sure not to do is add stuff like sugar, creamer, and such. Some people suggest using coconut oil but make sure that you factor it into your caloric intake.

One of the things you'll want to take into consideration is using some support supplements during your fast. They will help you ease your way into the fast and will provide additional nutrients during your fast. Consider something like magnesium and salt, which are ideal electrolytes. They will help you replenish your stores. Some fasters have sworn by grass-fed liver tablets which will help you by providing micronutrients. BCAAs or Branch chain amino acids will help to prevent the loss of lean tissue. Green powder is ideal for adding needed micronutrients. Omega 3 supplements will help too, so consider getting cod liver oil or algal oil.

Overall, fasting-mimicking is an excellent way to get the benefits of fasting while not putting as much stress on your body. You're doing the whole process of fasting, but you're still getting a form of nutrition and food. As you move forward with it, remember these three things: be kind to your body and if things seem like they're going south, don't hesitate to stop; set up your environment so that you're geared toward success with fasting; keep your calorie counts low and use the right supplements to stay within ketosis.

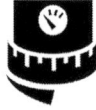

8

The Bonus Weight Loss of Autophagy

NOW THAT WE'VE explored the world of autophagy let's look more closely at how to use it to lose weight. To use the power of autophagy, you're going to have to follow a form of fasting. For those who are starting out, we'd strongly recommend the intermittent fasting method. You'll be able to eat a well thought out diet within a particular time frame every day, and for the rest of the day, you'll be in a fasting mode so that your body is burning the fat. Those who have used autophagy to lose weight are sometimes on high-fat diets for about 8 hours while for the remaining 16, their metabolism is getting to work breaking down and burning what they consumed before that. This will put you on a track that is simple but easy to follow so that you're able to get close to that figure you've wanted for forever.

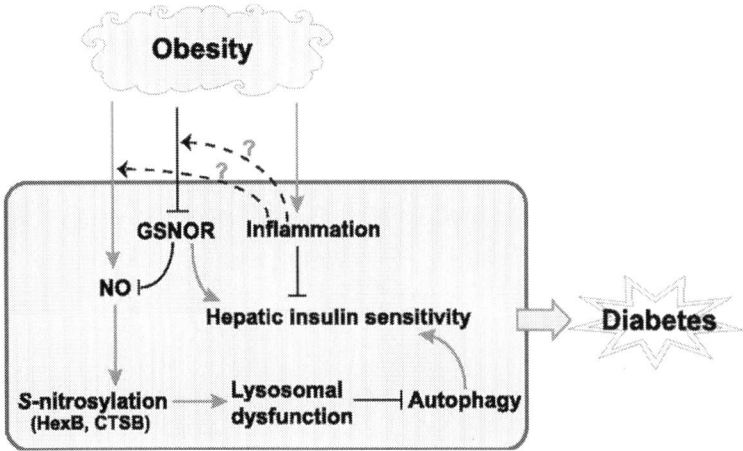

However, as we've noted, again and again, this isn't something you just do on your own and without help. You'll need to do research. This book has already given you a great start toward that. Find an expert to help you do other things such as plan meals, set which hours you'll be fasting (which will depend on your work and lifestyle), what workouts work for you, and what type of diet, if you so choose to go that route, will work for you. You'll also want to be sure that you're drinking enough water. Yes, we hear it all the time – drink more water, drink more water – that's because it's true, and it's especially true when fasting and wanting to lose weight. You'll want to speak to an expert on how much water your body will need to keep the autophagy going. Remember this: if you're not drinking enough water, your body will not flush the toxins being released. Then you're doing your body even more damage and further hindering your progress.

This all being said, go grab yourself a tall glass of water, and sit down and read the following stories collected from online from people like you. They have learned the benefits of autophagy and decided to share them with the world. Let them inspire you to stay that big step today!

———

FROM *MEDIUM.COM/PERSONAL growth*:

"Hi there 🙋🙂 My name is Sumaya and thanks to Intermittent Fasting (or IF for short), in 7.5 months I've dropped 50 pounds, 10.5% in body fat and 40 inches around my body. These results are entirely a result of if as I was unable to exercise for the first several months due to a fractured foot.

After college, I spent at least 5+ years in the overweight category (no thanks to bad habits, traveling and eating out) before spending another 5+ years in the obese category (no thanks to startup stress, late nights and even more work travel). I'm now officially in the normal weight category (according to my BMI).

I tried everything from Jenny Craig/Weight Watchers to going to the gym 4–5x a week to weekly meal prep. While I did see some results, I eventually couldn't keep up with it, and then yo-yo'd. IF has been the simplest and most manageable way I have found to improve my health (and stick with it).

This post is intended for my friends (and friends of friends) who have been following my health journey on Facebook, Snapchat or Instagram and have asked how to get started. Because the interest has been in the thousands (so amazing!), I've decided to share this information more publicly."

Note: To follow Sumaya's outline and tips in more depth, please go here. She goes over intermittent fasting in a personable way. Let's look at her online progress diary to see how it worked out for her. She notes that she used the Weight Gurus Digital Scale with smartphone tracking. That particular scale measured her weight, body fat, and muscle mass. The app is free, she says, and it showed her how her weight loss was trending. It allowed her to break down her goals into smaller milestone goals. This helped her predict, based on her current weight loss rate, at what point she would hit her targets. Her chosen style of intermittent fasting was what is called the "4:3 style." What this means is that she ate for four days during the week and fasted three non-consecutive days of the week.

THE FOLLOWING IS how she set her schedule up:

"SUNDAY: Eat Day // I eat as I normally would throughout the day, and I begin my fast at 9 pm PT (this means I stop eating or drinking anything with calories).

MONDAY: Fast Day // on fast days I only drink coffee, tea, non-caloric drinks and water (flavored sparkling water like La Croix has been awesome during fasting; my favorite is the Peach-Pear flavor). I add a little half & half in my coffee, and those are the only calories I consume on fast days. If/when I feel hunger pains on fast days, I drink a bottle/can of sparkling water, and that helps me get through the day.

TUESDAY: Eat Day // I break my fast at 9 am PT. I eat my full day of meals. The total calories I eat is my TDEE (total daily energy expenditure) range. I use this tool to calculate my TDEE:

https://tdeecalculator.net/index.php I start my fast again at 9 pm PT.

WEDNESDAY: Fast Day // Same as Monday.

THURSDAY: Eat Day // Same as Tuesday.

FRIDAY: Fast Day // Same as Monday & Wednesday.

SATURDAY: Eat Day // Same as Tuesday & Thursday.

SUNDAY: Eat Day // Same as Tuesday, Thursday & Saturday.

In summary: MWF = Fast Days, TuThSaSu = Eat Days. Repeat every week, and you will see and feel the difference."

For those who aren't a fan of her shorthand style, she does give you a more detailed outline of what her days were like:

"I start my fast at 9 PM and end the day after next at 9 AM, but these time frames can also be changed. Some of my friends prefer 7 PM/7 AM, 8 AM/8 PM, etc. to better accommodate their work/family schedule.

I have found that the 4:3 style fasts have worked well for my friends and I based on our work/life schedule and our personal health goals. I like that full day fasts feel like an on/off switch—I don't think about eating on fast days and on eating days if I happen to overeat, I don't feel guilty about it (since I'm eating at a deficit during the week). I find it more manageable to cut calories over a week (using the 4:3 style of IF) instead of every day (trying to eating less daily)."

"On Fast Days:

Having water on hand (especially sparkling water like La Croix) helps a lot

Let people you see often (friends, family, colleagues) know you're experimenting with IF. You'll be surprised how many people will work around your schedule, be supportive and take interest in IF.

If you need help getting through a Fast day, you can have up to 500 calories to eat without it technically considered breaking your fast. The 500 calories can be used as a crutch to get through the first few fast days. After week 2, you shouldn't need it.

If for some reason you do break need to break your fast (and eat more than 500+ calories), count that day as an Eat day and eat your full days' worth of calories (your TDEE). Don't try to fast the following day and just stick with your weekly schedule."

"On Eat Days:

I have found that eating high protein especially during my lunch and dinner meals keeps me better satiated on my fast days.

It's super important to EAT your full days' worth of calories since you are already eating at a deficit on your fast days. Do not skip meals or try to eat less."

"Intermittent Fasting can be challenging especially at the beginning which is why having support early on is important. I'm fortunate that my sister, brother and good friends all fast with me now (which makes the lifestyle easier).

I encourage you to introduce ID to a friend, family member or even colleague so that you can experiment with it together!"

What Sumaya's account tells us is that fasting and initially autophagy isn't as tricky as many newer people will assume it to be. She breaks down the way she successfully fasted so that anyone will be able to mimic her.

———

COMMITTING to our goals is difficult alone. We all want to share part of ourselves with others because it reminds us that we're human. One meaningful way we share parts of ourselves is through our stories. Why are they so important to us? Well, we desire to know that other people are dealing with what we're dealing with. We want to express ourselves. We have difficulties that arise in our lives. We become attached to these stories, wether they are happy, sad, and even full of pain. They become essential parts of our worlds.

Telling our stories is just the beginning. We tell them to release ourselves from them and watch them be like little children and grow and evolve beyond our minds. We share our stories to transcend ourselves. We want to learn about our history as humans, and many of us hope that in some capacity we can make a difference in the world with our stories. We listen to other accounts to broaden our perspectives. We want to see beyond the horizons of our minds. We want to act beyond a story because when it's stuck in our chests, it's locked there and we become prisoners of our own thoughts. Metaphorically speaking, it lets our spirit breath when we can finally open the cage in our chest and let the words flutter away.

Telling these stories also help to benefit future generations. Right now, we are living in the technology age where we can connect with many people around the world. It is easy for anyone to put their words out there in the world. Words are what we needed when we were learning about autophagy for the first time. Words that you need to get inspired to begin fasting today. Moreover, even as we write this, we made ourselves a part of the future, but we will be part of the past when you read this. Our stories are what connect the present and the past to the future. As intense as it sounds, sharing our stories and learning from them is a noble way to honor those who have put the building blocks for understanding autophagy together. Leaving this mark is a way for us to enlighten those who will come after us.

We all have many stories within us and even more powerful stories to tell in the future, especially after autophagy and fasting have changed your life!

The following stories are meant to be reassuring and to help you benefit from getting the opportunity to have their wisdom passed onto you. This exchange, the one between you the reader and they the writers, can be very impactful because as someone who is starting out, perhaps you feel that you need some help and guidance from someone real, something that goes beyond the "science talk." The key word in making such a big change is "resilience." This is strengthened with the understanding that we are all both learners and experts within the various paths of life. We all have something to share with one another. Resilience and change came from when we start to understand that words (and thoughts) can have power in them. We forget this power, and it is one of the reasons why hearing other's stories from their hearts is under-appreciated.

Perhaps you'll learn more about autophagy and about yourself after reading these narratives. Maybe they will clarify some of the more complicated scientific ideas that we've gone over in the book. Many people who have talked about making changes in their lifestyle on this scale have said again and again that pausing to tell their story, and reading about them from others is an excellent reminder of where they want to go. It is so easy to veer from the proverbial road.

With all this in mind, look to the following stories straight from the writers for inspiration and think about how your story will be added to theirs soon enough!

———

FROM: *www.ginstephens.com/success-stories.html*

Kim and Ryan Smith shared their success story!

"The most common feedback we get from others is that they can't believe our transformation, that we are unrecognizable, and that we don't look like the same people.

We don't feel like the same people, either. It's more than the 200 pounds we have lost. After struggling with food for decades (him since childhood, me since my mid-20s), we are finally FREE. We have gained and lost weight. We have tried numerous diets, separately and together. We struggled. We felt deprived. We gave up hope that there was a better way. During our 15-year marriage, we dealt with a lot of change in our extended family, our finances and our careers. Dysfunctional eating became the one stable constant in the center of our lives.

I found Gin's book, Delay, Don't Deny, in May of 2017 at a time when Ryan and I were following two separate diets, ones through which we'd both lost a fair amount of weight. I call it "semi-successful struggling," because although these plans had taken the weight off our bodies, we were still grappling with cravings, "cheating," and ultimately, we were once-again starting to regain weight. We read the book, began clean fasting daily, and suddenly everything clicked. The fasting felt amazing, our food tasted delicious, and we could eat what we wanted. Eating in the same pattern helped us to get aligned in many ways. The remaining weight melted away within months and maintenance feels so natural. We only delay, we do not deny.

We now live a life where the struggle is gone. The changes in us greatly transcend the physical. Peace and joy have replaced fear and angst - we truly feel FREE. Everything about our lifestyle now - the saved time and money, the freedom from cravings, the ability to eat intuitively and enjoy every bite of food - it all seems to too good to be true. But it isn't - it is true, it's real, and it is available for everyone who embraces the IF lifestyle. I am grateful to Gin and consider her a true mentor - not just with the weight loss, but in our new venture to write a book that tells this transformation story in full. You can follow our progress at fastingfeastingfreedom.com. Wishing you all a happy, healthy journey!"

Here is Amber from Indiana's success story!

"I began slowly gaining weight around 10 years ago. I attribute this a time of extreme stress which caused me to quit caring for myself physically. Before this, I had always been what most would consider thin. It took a few years for the weight gain to become visible to others, and even then, most would not have considered it extreme. It wasn't until about 2015 that it really became noticeable.

I rationalized my weight gain, however, and consoled myself with the comparison to others. On occasion, I would encounter a picture that I was not able to throw out, and I would be confronted with the truth. I had gone from wearing sizes 4-6 to wearing 12-14's at the height of my weight gain. I had no idea how much I weighed, as my scale had broken years before and I had never replaced it.

In the summer of 2017 I made a trip to Bed Bath and Beyond, and on a whim, I decided to step on one of their operating scales. Before I did, I guessed that at 5' 7.5" that my weight would be in the 160-pound range. I knew that wasn't great, but in my mind, I could justify it. So, I stepped on the scale, and it said 188.8 pounds. I stood in the store in front of two other women and wept.

In a moment of clarity, I decided to get it together and buy the scale. I went home and had a total pity party. "How could this happen? When did this happen?" I knew the answer to both questions. I had done all of it.

The next day I got up and resolved to fix the problem that I had created. I was the only one capable of digging myself out of the hole. I began by just watching what I ate, walking every day, and focusing on healthy fats and portion control. It wasn't long after that I began a HIIT workout three times a week. I lost weight with this approach, but an odd thing happened... I found that when I got up in the morning that I no longer wanted to eat breakfast. In fact, I resented being told that I must.

At some point on my Facebook feed, I started getting information about Intermittent Fasting from various sources. One that I remember suggesting that women should fast 12-14 hours, and then have their first meal. I dabbled with that for some time and felt great doing it.

It wasn't until November of 2017 that Delay, Don't Deny: Intermittent Fasting Support showed up on my Facebook feed. I was intrigued and joined the group. Within a day or two, I had purchased the book and read it in an evening. I've never looked back since.

Starting in November, I began fasting 16 hours a day. I quickly within a couple of weeks went to 19:5 and then shortly thereafter went to One Meal a Day or OMAD. It felt so natural and free. In the middle of December of 2017, my husband joined me in OMAD, and we are still OMAD to date.

Before IF I had lost 19 pounds. Since I began IF at the beginning of November 2017, I've lost an additional 31 pounds for a total of 50. My husband has lost 30. In addition to the weight loss, both of us have a renewed lease on life and an appreciation for each other. I no longer have to pick my clothes based on what I need to cover up, but rather what I should showcase. At 48, that is a definite WIN. :) My husband has found increased endurance for his physically demanding job as a builder at 57.

Neither one of us plans on ever going back to eating as we did before.

Intermittent Fasting is now our lifestyle.

Thank you, Gin for making this accessible and easy to understand! 🖤"

Here is Alex Boss's success story!

"I was one of those kids who could eat anything they like and still be skinny (I just grew taller instead, finally reaching 6' 4"). I was also into many sports (swimming, tennis, football). In my 20s, I cycled to work every day (over 100 miles a week), which meant putting on weight was still never an issue for me. I was used to eating what I liked and as much as I liked and still being slim, but in my 30s when my son was born, I found I was too tired to cycle in to work, I would eat sugary snacks just to pep me up for the afternoon (which of course just meant I crashed an hour later and turned to more high sugar snacks...). I slowly put on weight but then took action (no unhealthy snacking at work) and slowly lost some of it again; until, that is, my daughter was born. Again, the sleepless nights with a baby caused a bad diet, eating to stay awake at work, too tired and zero energy, and no free time to exercise. I gained several kgs. I had always been between 85kg and 88kg (187-195 lbs.), but I had gone up to 93kg (205 lbs.). Not massive, but I felt I had no control. My thighs started rubbing together as I walked. I thought there was no way 'back.' I had never been on a diet in my life, and everything I had heard told me that "diets don't work!" You end up weighing more. People told me that weight gain is what happens as you get older, as your metabolism slows you get the middle age spread, that's life...but that's not how I see myself, and that's not how I want to be. But what could I do?

I have a biology degree, so I began to read about the biomechanics of weight loss. I read about how hard it is and why people can't stick to diets - I read lots about metabolism and sugar, ketogenic diets, and then about insulin resistance and fasting...I watched documentaries and YouTube videos, which then led me to videos about fasting and the benefits. That's when I came across intermittent fasting, I could still eat for 8 hours a day and loses weight, build muscle, heal my body, and stop the all-day sugar rollercoaster. It seemed too good to be true! I started slowly, just missing breakfast and having black coffee (Yuk!!), then having lunch at 12 and eating normally, with dinner to finish at 8 pm. In the first couple of months I had hard days and easy days, but the more I did the clean fast, the easier it got (and the more I learned to love black coffee) and the more I enjoyed it. I found Gin and Melanie's podcast (www.ifpodcast.com) and then Gin's book and her support groups.

I eat two meals a day (TMAD), usually in an 8-hour window, and sometimes as low as 5 hours. Getting the feeling of being in Ketosis and knowing I am burning fat, knowing I am in control of my weight, and knowing that I am going to be eating a large satisfying meal later all felt great. I eat so well: bread, beer, pizza, chocolate, ice-cream, hamburgers, steaks, cheese, pasta, bacon! But the longer I did it, the smaller the quantity of food I wanted, and the healthier foods seemed so much more appealing. I am now 1.5 years in, doing IF every day (well most days). I am leaner now than I have ever been in my adult life (82kg) I am in control and I love this way of eating. It's so simple and easy to apply, and I even love my black coffee! (Cold brew in the summer.) I have signed up for a triathlon this August, and I am learning about being a fat adapted athlete.

I am looking forward to getting older, feasting on what I

want and staying in great shape with ease. It's all so simple: Delay, don't deny!"

Kela from South Carolina also shared her success story!

"I did it!!!! Today marks my 365th day of IF and the first time in my life I've had the willpower to focus on my own health and happiness.

I'm 5'9" and always been "big boned" with an obese/overweight BMI. My highest weight was 192lbs in October 2016, and I've lost less than 20lbs since starting IF a year ago. I've always weighed "a lot," but that doesn't make it any easier to still have a BMI in the overweight range despite my commitment to clean fasting since day 1. For many, that small amount of loss would be a reason to quit.

I've spent most of my adult life in a size 12/14 weighing a little more than I do now give or take. I started IF wearing size 10 jeans. This past summer I bought all new clothes in size 8. Now they are all too big. I had to buy smaller underwear for the first time in my adult life. Large t-shirts are too big on me for the first time in my adult life. That string bikini I bought as a joke...well, it's too big. I've run several races over the past few years, and all my running shorts/shirts are too big. I'm just about ready to commit to size 6 jeans...but not yet. I'm no longer the girl who is "large" everything. I weigh less than what is on my driver's license...and we all know that was a lie from the start. I am no longer the "biggest" person when in a group of people. If you have been this person without fail, you know how painful that is. IF has healed some of the autoimmune aspects of my hypothyroidism. I really do look younger! This is why we don't quit. This is why we trust the process.

I truly eat whatever I want during my window. I am REALLY good at delaying, knowing I don't have to deny. During the work week, I pretty much stick to OMAD. During the weekends, I have more of a window. We went on vacation this summer where I stuck to my window and had no weight gain. We went to Disney for a week where I stuck to an extended window and had no weight gain. This holiday season was the most relaxed I've been this whole year and the couple of pounds I gained (and will lose by the end of the week) were totally worth it. This flexibility and not restricting what I eat has been what helped me be successful. I'm sure I could lose more weight with more restrictions, but I can promise you I would have quite a long time ago. Besides, people don't see my scale, but they certainly see my figure. If only my face would get with the program and slim on up...

My food preferences have definitely been the biggest change since starting IF. I'm not opposed to cake and sweets, but I'm not as dependent on sugar as I once was. I used to NEED something sweet after eating, or I would get shaky. I struggled with hypoglycemia on a regular basis...but not once in the last 365 days, even when donating blood. I crave veggies and quality proteins. I started eating/craving real, quality cheeses for the first time in my life. The thought of wasting my one meal on fast food, boxed meals, or cheap sandwiches hurts my soul. When I do want sweets, I gravitate toward a specific taste rather than anything and everything in the pantry. Poor Little Debbie is lost without me. Despite trying everything, I haven't been able to adapt to black coffee, so

I open my window every day with a cup of sweet, creamy coffee as my own little "high five" for sticking with it.

I know this is long, but I hope this helps someone else stay the course. I've watched my mom diet since the day I was born. I grew up never knowing what full-fat salad dressings and non-diet sodas tasted like. I never understood why she couldn't love herself and see own beauty, in the same way, I loved her and thought so was beautiful. Then I became a mom, and those little punks did to my body what I did to hers. It became very hard to feel worthy or lovable. I dabbled in Weight Watchers, counted calories once, and took one diet pill (no thanks) but could never commit because I knew they didn't work. I'd watched my mom lose and gain and lose and gain my whole childhood. She has the willpower of steel, and I knew I wouldn't be able to measure up. But this...THIS WORKS. Maybe I haven't lost a lot of weight, but I have healed a very broken body and have patched up a much-damaged soul. This was for me. I can say, without a doubt, IF has become and will remain my lifestyle."

Sarah Morley also has a success story!

"I came across the Delay, Don't Deny Facebook page when I started looking into Intermittent Fasting back in July 2017. I was finding it increasingly more difficult to keep the weight off, even though I was eating fairly healthily and was running twice a week. I went on to buy Gin's book, and it just made so much sense. I started doing 16:8 at the end of July just before I went on holiday for two weeks. The week before my holiday I dropped about 4lbs. I did a bit of IF on holiday and when I returned I started doing 20:4 every day. During September, I was trying to keep to an LCHF (low carb high fat) diet and then started to add more carbs into my diet. I have been steadily losing weight, and my measurements are down each week. When I started looking into IF I was a UK size 14 and now in December I am a size 10. I have lost 16 lbs. to date and feel great. The support from the Facebook group has been immense and to see so many others having success with DDD just keeps me motivated. I've started upper body weight training over the last four months, just twice a week and I love it. I often work out in a fasted state, and I can see that my arms are shaping up and getting muscle definition. I can't believe how easy this way of life is and thanks to Gin for all her support, knowledge and encouragement. I introduced both my husband and my sister to IF and they are having great success. I love the freedom it gives me, and I no longer feel guilty about the foods I love to eat. I'm 47, and I'm back to being in better shape than I was in my 20's. The DDD lifestyle is for keeps!"

Add Terry DeGraw to the mix!

"Morbid obesity plagued me for 15 plus years. I used every excuse I could to justify eating: celebrate, happy, sad, holidays, even the death of my mom. I even told myself I'm fat and happy. That was one of the many lies I told myself about my weight.

I complained frequently about my weight, and a true friend suggested low carb. I made the decision to start after a vacation in April 2017. When I came home from vacation, I started immediately, and within a couple of weeks, I started feeling less bloated. That, in and of itself, was very motivating. By June I was down 25 pounds eating 2 boiled eggs for breakfast, 2 for lunch, and a small portion of meat and green vegetables for dinner. I never cheated, and I never snacked. I was and still am strict. In July I reduced my 2 breakfast eggs to 1 and replaced my 2 lunch eggs with a premier protein drink. By August I wasn't hungry for breakfast, so I started skipping it. I started doing some research and discovered intermittent fasting. I quickly realized I was fasting from dinner each evening until my protein drink at lunch.

Further research revealed OMAD (one meal a day). I stumbled upon Gin's books and her Facebook group. In September I started OMAD. To begin OMAD, I simply cut out the lunch protein drink, and suddenly I was living one meal a day, feeling so good and full of energy. I was instantly hooked. I lost 55 pounds eating low carb in 5 months, and I've lost an additional 37 pounds doing OMAD for 2 months.

My goal was to just be normal, so I set a goal of 150 when I started my journey at 237 pounds. I reached that goal with low carb and OMAD. Once I reached 150, I reset my goal for 145. Once I reached 145, I reset my goal for 137. I'm 5', and 137 pounds puts me in the normal category on the charts for my height. I have gone from women's plus size 20 stretch pants and a 3xl top to size 5 jeans and small tops from the juniors department. I'm still reeling, and sometimes I'm afraid it's a dream, and I may wake up fat. My husband has not joined me in OMAD. However, he eats low carb with me and has lost 46 pounds. We are happier as smaller people. It's been a great journey for us together. My new found revelation of eating to live versus living to eat has changed my life. I'm healthy and full of energy. I'll be 49 in Jan. of 2018, and I feel 30. If I had to say in a few words what I've learned from this journey, it would be to listen to my body and trust the process of clean fasting. It's given me my life back. #OMADNESS"

Natasha from Trinidad discusses her personal struggles and triumphs as well!

"Throughout my 30s I've had struggles with weight loss. I have tried lots of strategies, including the 1000 Cal and HCG diets, diet pills, brutal exercise regimens....you name it, I tried it in my quest to lose and keep off-the-shelf weight. In the end, I would regain all and more. Why? Because I love food, would eat whatever...whenever, and have the stuff that I restricted in abundance once I reach my goal of dieting.

In February 2017, I decided on a spiritual fast to adopt good eating habits. Yes, I sought God to deal with my problem. I decided that if my body is a temple of God, then I should treat it as such. I embarked on a stringent 21-day prayer and fast which started on the 1st day of the said month. During this time, I'd have no rice, flour, meat or sugar, and whatever I consumed I'd have before 6 am and after 6 pm each day. Nothing but water during the 12 hours. Most days I consumed just the evening meal due to work or being too lazy to get out of bed at 5 to prepare breakfast.

At the end of the 21 days, I had gone from 192 to 182 lbs.

I was ecstatic, and that prompted me to look up the benefits of fasting. It was then I discovered what I know now as Intermittent Fasting. Yes, God answers earnest prayers. I watched videos on YouTube and read posts on different sites. One day I searched Facebook for Intermittent Fasting, and it was a pleasant surprise to find so many groups on IF there. I eventually decided on Gin's OMAD (One Meal a Day) group, and again, that had to have come from God, because I've seen posts by "professionals," and frankly, they leave a lot to be desired. Finding Gin's OMAD group was the beginning of the end of yo-yo dieting for me. I had finally discovered a way to eat without denying myself the foods that I love and would binge on after denying myself for the sake of dieting for long periods of time.

It turned out that OMAD didn't suit my lifestyle, but 16:8 does. I eventually taught of the sister group Delay, Don't Deny, and that's my "sweet spot." Almost supernaturally, I came into possession of Gin's Delay, Don't Deny book, and it was definitely a great help. I still refer to it sometimes.

I love that I'm no longer a slave to neither food nor the scale. Now losing is fun because it's effortless. My window opens at 8 am and closes at 4 pm because I love breakfast. By the way that's another advantage of IFing; it's adjustable to suit your schedule and RIGIDITY ISN'T NECESSARY!!! Hey, I swear by this "way of eating.""

Lisa Simpson's story is quite compelling as well.

"I've never been able to do the normal diets - eating

disorder since I was a teen (binge/purge), thinking that was a great way to lose weight. Didn't happen. For me, there were good foods and bad foods. If I ate the good ones, I was ok. If I ate anything I considered bad, I felt this overwhelming urge to get rid of it. The weight kept going up - every 5 pounds I gained, I wished I was where I'd been 5 pounds ago. I had short periods of lower weight while doing Community Theater, nightly walking my dog and jazzercise.

I actually visited a friend year ago and saw she'd lost weight - she said she ate dinner only, whatever she wanted. At the time, that just sounded crazy to me, and I dismissed it - wish I'd paid better attention.

I cleaned up my diet while doing some research on living on a food-stamp budget. Less eating out, more eating at home. Joined a co-op and started getting lots of fruit and vegetables to play with.

In the spring of 2015, I ran my first ever 5k, and at the pre-race pasta party, Team World Vision was there and said they could take me from 5k to marathon in time for the Chicago marathon in October. For whatever reason, I believed them and signed up. I spent that summer training, along with some weight training to strengthen my legs. I thought all that running would HAVE to help me lose weight. I finished that marathon, very slowly. I only lost 10 pounds, which went right back on when I quit running.

In late 2016, I found IF (intermittent fasting) and OMAD (one meal a day). I remembered that friend I'd visited. I started in January 2017 at a weight of 172, wearing mostly size 14s.

I saw absolutely no loss per the scale for at least 3 weeks, but my belly was going away, and clothes were fitting looser. I did a 72 hour fast and dropped 5 pounds, sat there for a while; another long fast with a drop, and sat there - but then my body seemed to start to learn what to do.

I generally use a 4-hour eating window but have had some longer ones when something comes up. I don't restrict because that would make me obsess. No journaling, because that would also make me crazy.

It's now September 2017. I wobble between 146 -148, but my body looks completely different. I'm wearing anywhere from 4s to 8s in clothes. I'm sleeping well, my skin looks better, and I have tons of energy. I had a physical recently, and the doctor said all my lab tests look great - my HDL was so high it offset my high LDL.

IF and OMAD gave me back my life, a life with confidence and food freedom."

Brian from California also had some great successes.

"I discovered this way of life almost by accident. A friend of mine started a keto diet, and I thought it might be dangerous for him, so I started doing some research. Through the research, I discovered Dr. Fung's videos on YouTube and discovered OMAD (one meal a day) soon after.

I was already doing the old calorie in calorie out diet (had just started) and thought "I can do this and it is much easier."

I was at 265 lbs. at the time (April 2017). I had what I thought was bad knees and hips due to old age and, though a pretty avid bike rider, would tire easily. I had quit wearing jeans after being unable to button my 42 waists and had switched to full-time overalls.

Just a month into OMAD, I went to an outdoor concert wearing the jeans I couldn't wear before and was able to stand and dance like nobody was watching for 5 straight hours! Absolutely no pain at all in the knees or hips!

I quit weighing myself about a month ago (July 2017) and was down about 40 lbs. at that point. I currently am wearing a 38 waist jean, and they are getting looser! I haven't felt this good since my 20s, seriously. I am no longer easily winded when I ride and have cut 5 minutes off of my bike commute to work! OMAD has been a miracle to me, allowing me to enjoy food (which I do) without guilt. No calorie, fat grams, or carb grams to count. If there was, I wouldn't do it. Period. I tend to be the kid who would be up to the tree he was told to stay away from 5 minutes ago, and that inner rebel has persisted into middle age. Tell me I can't eat it and I will shove it into my pie hole while looking you right in the face, lol.

So, what do I do, you ask? I eat once a day. Period. I sit down to a meal, and when I am done, I am done until the next day with very few exceptions. What do I eat, you ask? Honestly, whatever I want. I have pasta, pizza, burgers, cheesesteaks, dim sum, Mexican food, Indian food, brats, salads, subs, steak, and potatoes, etc. Nothing, and I mean nothing, is off the menu. The only rule is clean fast. I drink a lot of coffee, water, and mineral water during my fast times. Do I "cheat" ever you ask? Yup, once every couple weeks or so. Usually, it is because of a social event (party, etc.), but occasionally just because my body screams FEED ME! Now, I do not call that cheating. I call it living life. No guilt, because it is what you do most of the time that counts, not what you do only once in a while. My body is proof it's working!"

Donna shared her personal story and makes known that when she talks about "WOE," she means "way of eating."

"Delay, Don't Deny changed my life. I have been a lifer when it comes to diets. Calorie restriction and the latest diet craze became my way of life. I always lost weight rapidly but quickly lost my mojo. My husband and I have 2 beautiful grandsons (3 and 7). Looking into their eyes made me realize that FAT SUCKS and I want to be healthy for me and for them. Huge revelation right?

A friend told me about Gin Stephens and her DDD book. Bingo--a plan was made. I started with 16:8 but quickly switched to OMAD (One Meal a Day) with a 1-hour eating window. Amazing discovery--the weight fell off. I do IF every day, coupled with vigorous exercise 7 days a week. I keep my carbs to 20 grams and my protein to 20% of my intake. I follow an LCHF (Low Carb High Fat) plan and have dropped 75 pounds in 18 weeks. Bye, double chin and puffy cheeks. Hello, cheekbones. Love this way of eating. Thank your Gin for motivating me. The boys thank you too."

Here is Helen Steinke's story!

"Hello, everyone! A little about myself. I am 54 years of age and a stay at home mom and wife. I am married to an awesome man who is very supportive of this WOE (way of eating). I have a son and a daughter who are both married, and two grandchildren. Before my complete hysterectomy in 2006, I was 150 pounds. After the surgery, my weight went up. I tried many things, including spending my winters in the gym and eating low-carb meals and denying myself all the foods I really love to eat, with very little success. As long as I kept on that plan, I could keep a few pounds off, but as soon as I would stop going to the gym, the pounds would come back on. My thought was that I will never be that skinny again, so I need to learn to accept that.

Well, thank goodness my sister Katie introduced me to if on December 27, 2016. When she explained this way of eating, my response was: no, that can't be. How can you eat everything you love and eat all those carbs and lose a lot of weight? Knowing my sister, she LOVES her salads and vegetables, and can pretty much live off of that stuff alone. I was very hesitant BECAUSE I LOVE MY CARBS.... and I thought her weight loss was because of her love for salads and vegetables. My thought was, what can it hurt? The worst that can happen is I wouldn't lose weight.

I made myself a promise that I would give it an honest try for three months, and if I didn't see results I would give it up, so I dove right in and started with 23 /1. My starting weight..... 180 lbs. At exactly 7 months later, my weight is 149 lbs. I wish I had taken measurements, but I did not. I can tell you that I am down in sizes: Dress - from a large, too small or medium. Pants - from 12 to 8 or 6. Tops - from a large to a small.

Now, for all you people that have to sit and watch your loved ones eat lunch, I understand how hard that is, especially in the beginning. I would make an awesome breakfast and lunch for my husband and had to smell the food I was cooking, and then to sit there and watch him eat while I was sitting there with my cup of coffee ... IT WAS TOUGH! There were times I wanted to eat but kept going back to that promise I had made to myself. For the first month, when my eating window opened, so did the fridge and pantry door, and I would stuff as much food as I could get in my mouth, and as fast as I could while I was cooking supper ... LOL ... and it was all carbs and junk food. For me, after my first week of IF, I realized I had lost weight. I couldn't believe it! Yes, it was a lot of water weight I'm sure, but I continued to lose weight after that. That was all the motivation I needed to keep going, and I knew I would never give up this way of eating.

My plan is to be 140 lbs. before I begin maintenance. I know I will get there because I'm not giving up this way of eating ... I AM A FASTER FOR LIFE! For me, the weight came off fairly fast for the first four months, but the last two months have been very slow. For all of you that think it will not happen or is not happening anymore, it will! Keep at it: it's a lifestyle change. All I can tell you is ... DON'T GIVE UP! Nobody can take the weight off of you but yourself. Make a promise to yourself, and keep it. Something I heard a lot during this process from my sister is ... TRUST THE PROCESS! So I am telling all of you to do the same. When times get tough, find someone you can talk to for support and help you through the hard times. For me, it was Katie and all my sisters. So, thank you, girls, for being there and helping me through this. I couldn't have done it without you!!! GIN said it best... I DESERVE TO BE SKINNY ... that, my friends, has stuck with me. And for all of you that are struggling, tell yourself you want to be the next success story ... I can't wait to hear it!!! Thank you, Gin, for sharing your success story, and thank you for all the research and hard work you are doing for all of us and for sharing this awesome way of life with all of us."

Here is Terri's story.

"I've been trying to lose weight for the past 20 years. I've tried pretty much every diet out there. Spent about 10 years trying and failing at Carb Addicts Diet and Atkins. I just thought I was an utter failure because I couldn't stay away from the carbs. I felt horrible when I was sticking to low carb as I should be. I was pre-diabetic, had high blood pressure, and was starting to have trouble just getting around. My highest weight was 299. I lost and regained the same 50 lbs. over and over and over again. I had pretty much given up hope and resigned myself to just being sick and fat forever when for some reason the OMAD (One Meal a Day) Facebook page was advertised on my feed. I checked it out and then purchased The Obesity Code and read it in one sitting. I didn't think I could do the long fasts like Dr. Fung talked about in the book so I pretty much put it away. The next day out of curiosity I went back to the OMAD page, read Gin's book, and decided what do I have to lose, and I tried it. 7 months later I'm down 55 lbs. in total. My blood pressure is normal, my A1C is normal, and I feel great! First time

I've ever in my life felt in control around food. And I eat anything I like even CARBS! :D I've never ever stuck to anything this long. I intend to do it for the rest of my life.

100% FAITH IN DELAYING, NOT DENYING, & I AM PROOF OF ITS SUCCESS!

Today marks one month of intermittent fasting for me!! I have lost 16 pounds and a couple inches!

I was very fortunate to have always been a healthy weight most of my life. I just turned 34, and after having baby #3, I also got diagnosed with Hashimoto's about a year ago on top of having a baby. This really packed on the pounds for me.

I have never had to worry about food. I've always been able to eat what I wanted, as much as I wanted and when I wanted and never gained an ounce. If anything, I would lose weight. It was awesome. This gave me an excuse to love food even more. I loved me some Big Mac meals and lots and lots of soft drinks and high-calorie sugary Starbucks drinks. I had no self-control and would eat like a pig to my heart's content and still manage to wear a teeny bikini.

Fast forward to present day --if I do so much as even look at a Snicker's bar, I gain ten pounds. So, imagine how hard it is for someone who has become addicted to fast food/junk food/sugar and never had a limit....then now, where it's almost as though I'm coming off of a drug like I'm legit rehabbing! It's really freaking hard!

I have tried hundreds of diets and have failed every single one of them!! Dieting is hard! It's not practical, and it's boring! Not to mention, pure punishment!

I found the Facebook group, and thanks to Gin Stephens and her amazing book, I have fallen in love with DDD (Delay, Don't Deny) and OMAD (One Meal a Day)!!! It's the BEST thing that has ever happened to me!!

In 30 days, I have lost 16 pounds and 2 + inches. My skin is clear and glowing. The only cravings I get now are to exercise and I legit love my coffee black now!! (If you would have told me a month ago that in 30 days I'd be drinking my coffee black, I would have laughed in your face!) I have complete control over my appetite by enjoying large scrumptious meals, sometimes a plate of nachos or pizza, sometimes a spinach salad. My body tells me what I need and how much of it I need when I need it, and the best part of all, my body now tells me exactly when to stop eating. I no longer stress about food all day, I don't worry about calories, and I've saved a bunch of time and money by switching to OMAD.

The family members and friends who were stoning me for doing IF are now asking me for my guidance to start this way of eating.

I have never felt more in control of my life, and I have never felt healthier than I do right now! If you aren't DDD'ing, then you really don't know what you're missing out on!! This is my new life. I will never go back!!!"

A person who goes by the name of "The Awakening" shared their story too.

"I started dieting in 1968 when I was 14 years old. I have counted calories on various diets. I've counted carbs on the Marine's Diet when I was 18, then later on the Atkin's diet and recently on the New Atkins diet. I have counted points on the Weight Watcher's Diet a couple of times. Plus there have been many fad diets I have tried. I have always lost some weight only to gain it all back and then some. I discovered intermittent fasting last summer and started doing it every day on August 1st, 2016. I fast 19 -22 hours every day and have a 2 to 5-hour daily eating window. I've lost 41 lbs. so far and 8 1/2 inches in my waist. There are no words to express how happy and thankful I am now. I no longer count anything. I'm 62 yrs. old but feel like I'm 30. I take no medication, sleep like a baby and have so much energy that sometimes I don't know what to do with myself. I will live this lifestyle always!"

Brian tells us about how thankful he is for the change in his life!

"Here is a little story of why I'm so thankful for this way of life. In January, I began the task of seeking weight loss through bariatric surgery. I had tried everything. Diets failed, didn't have time to work out, and my body ached all the time. I had diabetes and hypertension.

A friend at work started telling me about fasting and how wonderful it was. I started researching to prove him wrong, and I couldn't. Bought the books, decided to give this a try and see what happens. My surgery was scheduled for July 20th. I had to attend 6 meetings with the dietitian, meetings with the physical therapist, and meetings with the doctors. Insurance wants to see if you are serious about weight loss, so you have to lose some kind of pounds for them to approve covering the cost. I did everything expected of me.

I started at the end of January - beginning of February with IF. Moved to OMAD (one meal a day) at the end of Feb. I have visited Paris, Chicago, and Chattanooga and eaten a lot of food for my one meal a day. I have gotten so much energy that I have stopped our lawn service as I cut the grass now. I have stopped paying for car washes since I wash my car and the wife. I stopped paying for a gym membership as I have an exercise bike, free weights, and a bunch of work to do at home. So, if getting healthy is about a lifestyle change - this has definitely changed the way I live and my mentality when it comes to food. I tend to look at food more as fuel and not a task I have to complete ("eat everything in sight - you are hungry Brian!").

Today was my final visit with my dietitian. Being down 38 lbs. since I started, I have decided to cancel my surgery. I have until the end of the year to change my mind, but.... if I think about it, the lifestyle I live now is working and well worth it. I have improved my life for the better. My house looks good, cars look good, and I look good, the bank account looks good (not spending a lot of money on food). My blood sugar is now in the range of pre-diabetes. My body feels cleaner, not getting pains and aches I use to get. I am not at my goal weight, but I am at my goal mindset. It was okay to love food, but don't let it control you; become an active member in your life and stop being lazy, and enjoy the life you live.

Many thanks to Gin and everyone in the OMAD FB group. It feels as if I've been reborn. I know I may not lose as fast as some, but all things considered, the future looks amazing. I wanted to reach my goal weight this year, but it may take another year, and that's perfectly fine with me. Life is about the journey and not the destination, so I'm letting the window down and enjoying the breeze, knowing I'm on the right path to success!"

Let's take a look at Kate's story.

"I've struggled with my weight for my whole life. I just kind of dealt with it until I was in 8th grade, at which point I decided to jump on the low-fat trend that was so popular in the early 90s. And it worked! I lost 80 pounds, rejoiced at the fact that I was finally thin and "normal," and then promptly put it all back on when I went back to eating "normally" again.

The weight slowly crept up and up over the years. I went up and down here and there. I tried to exercise and various fad diet plans, with minimal success, and ultimately I found myself at my highest weight of 273 pounds in 2015. In fact, I don't even remember being that heavy (I think I blocked it out), but I know it's true because it was logged into my fitness tracker at that point.

I started out my current weight loss journey doing a low carb/ketogenic diet in the spring of 2016. I had heard about keto from a friend who touted its effectiveness. I read up on it and started eating that way, and it was indeed effective, but I couldn't shrug off this feeling that I was still a slave to my weight. Sure, I could eat all the bacon I wanted, but I couldn't feel free to celebrate with a piece of birthday cake with my family or a glass of wine with friends. I had this constant anxiety that one molecule of dreaded carbs would erase all my hard work. I could never feel totally "normal" eating low carb. It wasn't a feasible lifestyle change for me, because it didn't fully allow me to live.

Luckily a friend of mine (the same friend who introduced me to keto, actually) told me to look up Intermittent Fasting. I did a little research online, which lead me to Gin's site and Facebook group. Before interacting at all in the group, I purchased her book, read up, and then got started. It's been an absolute game changer. Not only am I slimming down with ease, but I have incredible energy and confidence, my cravings for unhealthy foods has greatly diminished, I drink tons of water, and I no longer have anxiety about eating with other people. I no longer have to worry that I won't be able to find something I can eat at restaurants or parties. I no longer have to limit the types of meals I can make with my fiancé (bless his heart, he gave up a lot of yummy carbs at one point in time). Intermittent fasting has truly given me something I never thought I'd have: Freedom!

I am currently at my first goal weight, having lost almost 100 pounds! The next step is to keep on being an awesome IF'er, hit the gym to get svelte, and keep spreading the word to others who are struggling with their weight! This is a lifestyle everyone should be aware of. Thanks, Gin!"

Here is Sharon H. from North Carolina's story.

"My journey for me started last summer. I was at our pool when I started talking to a friend about losing weight. She told me about intermittent fasting...I listened....being very skeptical. She said I will add you to this group on Facebook. I started reading up on it and thought to myself what I have to lose!! So on July 13th I woke up and weighed myself...235 pounds!!! That was my starting day. I wrote my weight on the calendar and grabbed me a bottle of water. I jumped straight in with my five-hour window being from 4 to 9. The only major thing I did was quit drinking sodas. I still drink my sweet tea but only in my window. I drink strictly water until my window opens. I still eat whatever I want!! Cheeseburgers, pizza, pasta, and chocolate!! Now I don't eat as much as I used to, but I still get to enjoy my favorite foods.....which is absolutely wonderful!!! This way of life has been the best thing to ever happen to me!! Now my weight didn't drop right off in a couple of weeks, but from July 13th until now I have managed to lose 95 pounds!! Which still shocks me.....it has seemed way too easy? I haven't deprived myself of anything I enjoy eating!! I am 42 years old and feel better than I did when I was 30!! My body doesn't ache anymore, I am not tired all the time, and I feel great about myself!!"

Let's hear from Dave!

"My One Meal a Day Intermittent Fasting Journey started on January 3, 2017. On New Year's Eve, I was at 283 pounds, had high cholesterol, high blood pressure, and elevated enzymes on my liver. I felt bad and was tired of being me.

I always noticed how I was never hungry naturally until

around 2 pm every day, so I decided I would try eating just dinner and also starting looking to see if anyone else did something crazy like this to lose weight and get healthier.

I found Gin's book through a search on Facebook and joined her page (which I love), and the bought the book Delay, Don't Deny. After reading it and following all the tips and directions I began to change, and change for me came fast. Now only 3 months later all of my blood work came back normal last week! I am down 37 pounds and plan on dropping 35 more. I have a new way of life; it happens once a day."

Listen to Nick's testimonial!

"My testimonial is lengthy so if you prefer the cliff notes version: I was 235 lbs. in 2008 and 180 lbs. today in 2017; 25 lbs. of the loss is 100% attributed to intermittent fasting and one meal a day, which occurred over a two month period. I have never known such an effortless way of eating which adds countless health benefits and a new relationship with food.

Now for those who wish to know more, here we go. In 2004, I ended a 20-year relationship with the love of my life: Crystal Methamphetamine. As is the case with many recovering addicts, I replaced one addiction with another, food. Between 2004 and 2008 I went from 185 lbs. to 235 lbs., for a total of 50 lbs., all of which was fat. Not only was I looking horrible, but I began to have G.I. issues; it was time for a change. After some soul searching, the first thing I did was to become a vegetarian in 2008. This was as much for animal welfare as it was for my health. I still wasn't eating properly, and it would take some time before I stopped consuming processed fake meat products, which are filled with soy and a ton of multisyllabic chemicals, as my primary source of food.

In 2010 I watched Fat, Sick and Nearly Dead and incorporated juicing into my diet. Juicing helped me not only to lose about 10-15 lbs., but I also learned to enjoy the taste of fresh fruits and vegetables. After about 6 months of juicing, I decided to stop wasting so much food and just eat the whole thing; I was throwing away all the nutrient-rich fiber and pretty much just drinking sugar water. Now I was preparing my own meals made from fresh produce, but I was eating 3-4 times a day. At this point, I was introduced to a program that eliminated all flour and sugar from my diet. This was by far the most painful and restrictive program I had ever encountered. I had great success with this, but as time would prove, it was unsustainable. I found a post from Facebook 2012: "Target weight of 180 reached today! Highest weight was 235. Bounced between 218 and 235 for several years. Last year cut out flour and processed foods and sugar; the past five months I've been on a mostly vegan diet; cutting out the dairy really helped as well as an s### load of exercise." So reaching 180 lbs. I had become vegetarian on a mainly vegan diet and had also eliminated all flour, sugar and processed foods. I remember 2012 and 180 lbs. as being jubilant, but also that it was such an arduous process and I certainly was never satisfied with the food I was eating and always seemed to be hungry. I was exercising for 90 minutes a day at the gym; to reach this point was a huge effort and in hindsight, destined to fail. As with all calorie restricting diets, this was completely unsustainable, and within a year I had binged on flour and sugar to the point of reaching 200 lbs.

This was when I learned about Intermittent Fasting from Dr. Joseph Mercola's Facebook page. I loved the science behind this concept and in 2014 implemented. A 16:8 schedule which; I eventually dropped down to a 19:5. By June 2014, I reached an unprecedented 177 lbs. by keeping a five-hour window, but I was also denying myself any processed sugar, and I was eating a lot of raw vegetables; again not very satisfying or sustainable. July 2014 my husband underwent brain surgery, and I took off time from work to care for him. At this point IF flew right out the window and I returned to the dreaded 3 meals a day. Slowly, at first, 5 lbs., 10 lbs., 15 lbs.; the same pattern emerged so that by the spring of 2016, I had reached 205 lbs.

By December 2016 something finally began to shift in me. I don't remember where I first ran across the idea of one meal a day, but I started watching some YouTube videos on the idea. Then on December 24th I told my husband what I was considering doing and asked for his support; he gave it without question. Christmas Day 2016 was my first attempt at one meal a day. I chose a one hour window between 10:30am and 11:30am. At work, there was a Christmas dinner for all employees. Which was difficult, but I passed; day one was a success! After finding that I didn't wither away from starvation, I decided that if I were going to attempt this as a lifestyle, I would need to establish this as a habit: I committed to OMAD for 30 days. This proved to be a wonderful tool, and I recommend to all beginners to commit to a timeframe to establish this as your new normal. This was also when I searched Facebook for a community of like-minded people, and fortunately, the first group I found was Gin Stephens' group, One Meal a Day IF Lifestyle. For a former twelve-stepper which is not very fond of groups, this group has made all the difference in the world and is a huge part of my success. I have never known such a supportive and inspirational group of people. After being part of this community for only a few days, I decided to purchase Gin's book: Delay, Don't Deny, which I found to be an excellent book especially for someone just beginning this lifestyle. Today I am 5 pounds away from an arbitrary number of 175 lbs. I'm not sure what my actual weight will eventually be; I'm waiting to see what this body decides. Every day I am learning to listen to this body because it knows exactly what it needs and how much it should weigh. There truly is no reason I can find, not to continue this lifestyle and way of eating; there are so much freedom and empowerment with this way of life. February 14, 2017."

Here is Laura from Bristol, UK sharing her story.

"I am a mother to 3 young boys. Before I had children, I had always struggled with my weight, and I was what people call a yo-yo dieter, putting on weight and losing alternatively within months. I had 2 children 15 months apart, and my weight rocketed. I was introduced to fasting through the 5:2 diet and lost about 30 lbs. Then, I came across intermittent fasting: One Meal a Day and Fast-5. It was a concept I thought I could follow after researching about it all.

Just before starting this new way of life I found out I was

expecting my third bundle of mayhem and mischief. During my final pregnancy I put on over 4 stone (56 lbs.), and that weight wasn't going anywhere after having little man. 3 months after my son's birth I decided enough was enough, and I found Gin's page. I thought, "Let's go for it!" Although I am a very quiet member of the Facebook group, I am on it daily. The support has been amazing.

I started doing IF, and now just over 2 years later I am over 68 lbs. down and only 5 lbs. away from a target that I haven't hit for many years. I truly believe IF what has got me there is. Friends and family have always been skeptical, and of course, I hear the usual remarks of "starving yourself" and "it's not healthy." I now just let them have their opinions, but no one can deny after seeing my before, and after that, it doesn't work.

I feel so blessed to have found this new way of life. Some days are harder than others, and when life throws you a curve ball, you have to resist falling back to old habits. I know I feel healthier, sleep better, and have more energy. I am actually starting to enjoy seeing my reflection again in the mirror, and not avoiding them at all costs, which is what it has been for the last 5 years

ANYONE CAN DO THIS!

Never thought I would ever write a success story. I never succeed on any diet before (and I've tried so many.) After giving birth to my three kids, I was about 80 kg (176 pounds), and I started one meal a day (OMAD) after I was proposed to in October of 2016. I thought it would be hard... but it's the easiest thing I've ever done! Only giving up on my diet soda and drinking my coffee black was a hard thing to do ;-) I've lost 32 pounds (16 kg) so far without working out and I eat whatever I like with my family within my window (mostly 3 or 4 hours). Since OMAD I feel like I've escaped out of diet prison :) I can do this for the rest of my life. So happy I've found OMAD, and the book really made sense, I learned so much from it!"

The following story can be found at

http://foodcanwait.com/home/my-weight-loss-journey-intermittent-fasting/

From Mimi titled "Intermittent Fasting: My Weight Loss Journey"

"Maybe you'll recognize yourself in these paragraphs. Before I began practicing daily intermittent fasting, my day consisted of constant eating. I would often delight in a morning cup of coffee, hot chocolate or tea with cream and sugar. Before lunchtime, I would likely have some kind of snack – sometimes a nutritious one like grapes or an apple, and sometimes a not-so-nutritious snack like potato chips, a donut or cookies.

By lunchtime, I was ready to eat again and would likely grab a meal from the nearby cafeteria – a sandwich, maybe a salad, and on Fridays, probably an order of fried fish. In the afternoon it was time for another snack to hold me over until I got home. During dinner time I would almost always have seconds, sometimes thirds, and late at night (I'm a night owl) I would snack again on sweets like homemade cookies or bread and/or something savory like nuts, cheese or chips.

Although I enjoyed vegetables like zucchini, broccoli, and

cabbage, my favorite foods were white rice, bread, and beans. I never got tired of those and could, and often did, eat them daily. I didn't indulge in fast food that often, but even when I cooked at home, there was little concern for neither whether my protein of choice was fried, baked or stewed nor the amount of fat, carbs, and calories I was consuming.

In short, I ate whenever and whatever I wanted to eat.

This eating pattern repeated itself over and over again, day after day and along with a mostly sedentary lifestyle working in an office, eventually resulted in my weighing 237 lbs. by June 30th, 2014. I knew it wasn't healthy to eat the way I did, but I felt unable to control my appetite even after trying just about every natural appetite suppressant I'd heard of – Sensa, garcinia cambogia, raspberry ketones, and others.

I had tried dieting many times in my life and lost 20, 30, and even 40 pounds on occasion only to gain it all back, and then some. But now I was almost afraid to lose weight for fear of the initial weight-loss only leading to being even heavier in the end. I wasn't fully aware of what I was doing to my body during the surges of calories I was feeding it; and, after a while, I didn't care much. After all, I didn't have diabetes, hypertension, or any major disease and I wasn't on any medication. What was there to be concerned about?

I hadn't always had such a nonchalant attitude about my weight. In 2004 I had lost 40 pounds on the Atkins diet and kept it off for two years only to gradually gain it all back within a year of being off the low-carb wagon. I began to think I should just accept being fat.

Obesity isn't just a cosmetic concern. It increases your risk of diseases and health problems such as heart disease, diabetes, and high blood pressure. -The Mayo Clinic website

Later that year, a visit to my doctor for a complete physical confirmed my relatively good health; but, he urged me to lose weight. He told me that at this time in my life – my forties – I was at a critical stage during which obesity greatly increased the odds of acquiring a major health condition within the next several years.

At that moment I thought back to my parents. My dad was diagnosed with diabetes in his mid-forties. My mom was diagnosed with hypertension in her 40's. There was no denying the significant probability of my going down the same path if my lifestyle didn't change.

Still, I didn't know how to do it. I'd tried low-carb dieting as well as low-fat diets with moderate exercise; but despite losing some weight with both, I could never seem to stick to either regimen in the long term. Then, shortly after that physical, a seemingly unrelated activity led to a complete lifestyle change for me.

Although I am not a Muslim, I had always been curious about fasting for Ramadan and admired the commitment and discipline needed to go without food or drink from sunrise to sunset for 30 days. I expressed my curiosity to a few of my Muslim co-workers, and they encouraged me to try it. My reasons for exploring Ramadan fasting were not religious, but rather psychological and spiritual. Did I have the self-discipline to subject myself to a period of mindfulness and self-reflection, setting aside a routine of comfort and ease to foster a greater sense of gratitude? That's the question I asked myself as I thought about committing to the 30-day fast.

As the time drew near to start, I was ready to quit my experiment before it began. I recall being scared, nervous and anxious to go without food; but that alone told me that I needed to do it. My co-workers didn't pressure me at all, but I felt a responsibility to at least try it. Still, by the time the start of Ramadan came, I hadn't fasted and didn't intend to do so. That is until I happened to watch an episode of Naked and Afraid.

As I watched the contestants spend weeks foraging for clean water and food sources much like our ancient ancestors had to do, I suddenly felt no better than a spoiled child unwilling to give up her lollipop. Certainly, I could survive less than a day without food or water. After all, if I changed my mind, nourishment was always within arm's reach.

With so much fear and anxiety before starting the fast, I hadn't expected to last a day, but to my surprise, not only did I last to the end of Ramadan, but the longer I fasted, the easier it became. What's more, I had indeed learned a lot about myself and developed a tremendous appreciation for access to clean water and nutritious foods — something I will never take for granted again.

After feeling so good, both physically and mentally, from the effects of fasting during Ramadan, I began exploring the health benefits of fasting and discovered intermittent fasting (IF). I had not fasted for Ramadan to lose weight. As a matter of fact, I had expected to gain weight from feasting at the end of the day. Like many people, I believed one should eat several small meals a day and never skip meals and that doing so was counterproductive to weight-loss. But, I had lost 8 pounds by the end of that month and felt exceptionally energized and in control of my hunger. There were clearly benefits to fasting, and as I researched more, I learned that there were even more pros than I had first imagined – one of them being weight loss.

I began fasting on June 30, 2014. At that time I weighed 237 lbs. That's a lot of weight on any woman, but on my 5'5"frame it was dangerous. As of the writing of this post (a little over three months later), I am 22 lbs. lighter and still working towards my goal of being at a healthy body mass index (BMI).

So far, daily intermittent fasting, a low-carb (non-ketogenic) diet a healthy diet focused on nutritious home cooked food, and 30 minutes of walking daily have enabled me to lose weight at a moderately steady pace.

Stay tuned. And to my fellow fasters, stay strong. We can do this!

All the best,

Mimi"

Mimi's journey didn't stop there. She gave her readers updates to give her journey even more of a spherical perspective.

"Update! Today is March 25, 2016, and it's been about a year and a half since I began my journey with daily intermittent fasting. As of today, I've lost 73 lbs. – down from 237 lbs. to 164 lbs. today. Although I haven't measured inches consistently, I know I've lost several as I've gone from a size 18 to a size 10.

After hitting the 50-lb weight-loss mark in June of 2015, I plateaued for over four months until I began incorporating the Five Bite Diet along with Fast-5. Within that week, I broke my plateau and over the course of a few months lost 24 lbs. Unfortunately, I gained some of that weight back after returning to Fast-5 alone; however, it did help me break a plateau and eventually I began losing again. I'll be sticking to Fast-5 alone for the remainder of my journey to my goal weight of 135 lbs. and a healthy BMI of 22.5. I recently began incorporating a plant-based diet into my fasting regimen, and so far I feel great!

At this point, fasting has become a solid habit for me, and I'm very comfortable with sticking to my 5-hr window. I'm excited to think that is the year I achieve my goal and begin maintenance."

———

YOUR LIFE IS ABOUT to change, and the best way you can acknowledge this is to think about and begin creating your story. Telling your story is a bit of a spiritual venture because it is the chance for us to get to the heart of who we are as individuals. Listening to other's stories is one thing, and creating your own is another. Doing so will be one of the most rewarding and fulfilling interpersonal experiences you've had. It is now your turn to empower yourself and others who will come after you by getting to a stronger, more intimate understanding of what this change will be for you and why it's so important and why you even got on this journey in the first place.

When you're creating your story, you're tapping into something that is universal and ageless. It is something that has been experienced by humans since the beginning of our collective existence. It connects us to our roots and offers us a long common heritage. Sociology tells us that we do so, on four different levels: the philosophical level, the spiritual level, the sociological level, and the psychological level. Consider it like a spiral that's moving toward the inner self. On the outer most part, we are telling the story at the universal level. We all want to connect with one another and feel like we're a part of something bigger. It is what inspires us to rise again with the sun (or the night sky for you night owls out there). From here comes the spiritual space, or where the mystery of life beckons for us to answer. This is where we feel and understand life through stories on a level that perhaps words can't quite explain, the gray area where faith and the metaphysical dwell.

Further inward comes with the world outside the self. This is where we continuously reach out; perhaps it's the reason why you picked up this book. You want to see what other people have said about autophagy. You think that it can change your life, but you want to know how it will do so. What makes it so important? What is it that has everyone's tongues wagging? Is it more than just another fad? Is it as simple as those who understand it said it is?

Finally, we come to the center of the spiral – ourselves, or the psychological. This is where is going to be the most challenging and this is where your story will come in handy. Without yourself, there is no fasting, there is no lifestyle change, and there is no new chapter in your story.

It's time to take what these people have given you and be a guide yourself. These stories, like yours, are guided by the universal and ageless prototype that guided the sacred and traditional stories of past generations. Your story will have the same enduring fundamentals, motifs, and archetypes. It will remind yourself and others that there is a way to get through the twists and turns of the paths of our lives. There is no real beginning, middle, and an end to a story. There are instead many beginnings, the muddled parts, and then a resolution. Moreover, this where we want you to be on your journey.

As you begin your journey, we'd like to leave you with Dr. Yoshinori Ohsumi's speech as he accepted the Nobel Prize in 2016. You can watch it here if you want to hear it from the man himself.

"I wish to thank to the Nobel Assembly at Karolinska Institute and Nobel Foundation for awarding me the most prestigious prize in science, the Nobel Prize, in the category of Physiology or Medicine. I'd also like to congratulate this year's other recipients. It has been lovely meeting everyone during this very enjoyable week, and it is an honor to stand among such esteemed people.

I am just a basic cell biologist who has been working with yeast for almost 40 years. I would like to take this opportunity to note my appreciation for the many lessons and wonderful gifts from yeast – perhaps my favorite of all being sake and liquor.

My research career focused on autophagy, which is a major process of recycling and degradation of proteins within cells. Life is maintained by a delicate balance between continuous synthesis and degradation. I found that degradation is just as important as a synthesis for the maintenance of dynamic biological systems like the body.

My group's contribution was to find the molecular underpinnings of autophagy. Autophagy is now exploding into one of the most intensely studied topics in biology. While our contribution is fundamental, it is pleasing that many researchers are now studying its relevance in health and trying to conquer a range of diseases. There is no greater satisfaction as a scientist than seeing your ideas and efforts transform a field of research, and I am as happy as I could be. I will finish by acknowledging the fortune, a large number of excellent collaborators, indispensable grant support and caring family that brought me here tonight. Thank you again all for this wonderful opportunity."

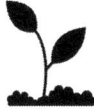

Afterword

Research is telling us more and more each day that autophagy, which was once just considered a humble little maintenance pathway, may be the key to preventing metabolic dysfunction and illnesses. Its utility can differ depending on where it is in the body, which makes autophagy a blossoming scientific wonder that can be the gateway to future treatments within science and medicine. All the contributions leading up to the 2016 Nobel Prize are now widely recognized by the masses, and this helps us understand just how essential autophagy is to our lives. The usefulness arguably goes beyond any other type of "fad" that we've seen come and go in the blink of an eye. To improve our understanding of autophagy, we must continue to support further research in the coming months and years. This is even more critical because, as we've seen when discussing the benefits of autophagy with cancer treatment, it is still a double-edged sword for us. We don't want to reverse what ground we've already trodden. There have been some many questions answered about autophagy, but there are still so many other questions that are still yet unanswered. However, with the persistence of more research and with the help of those of who have learned and utilized the wonders of autophagy, we will be able to overcome the concerns that currently keep us from completely understanding of what autophagy is fully capable.

———

Thank you for making it through to the end of *AUTOPHAGY: Extended Water Fasting is the Powerful Secret of Healing and Anti-Aging using Your Body's Natural Intelligence.* Let's hope it was informative and able to provide you with all of the tools you need to attain your goals whatever they may be.

The next step is to consult an expert and to have a meaningful discussion about how to start inducing autophagy and begin fasting in your life today.

Finally, if you found this book useful in any way, a review on Amazon is always appreciated!

More References

For more information on autophagy and the on-going research revolving around it, please visit the following sites:

- https://www.ncbi.nlm.nih.gov/pmc/articles/PMC2990190/
- http://genesdev.cshlp.org/content/21/22/2861.full.html
- http://science.sciencemag.org/content/330/6009/1344
- https://www.novusbio.com/research-areas/autophagy
- http://www.biochemj.org/content/475/11/1939
- https://www.annualreviews.org/doi/abs/10.1146/annurev-immunol-042617-053253
- http://journals.plos.org/plosbiology/article?id=10.1371/journal.pbio.2002864
- https://www.ahajournals.org/doi/abs/10.1161/circresaha.108.188318
- http://www.scielo.br/scielo.php?script=sci_arttext&pid=S0104-42302017000200173
- https://ard.bmj.com/content/74/5/912
- https://www.jci.org/articles/view/37948

- https://academic.oup.com/advances/article-abstract/9/4/493/5055944?redirectedFrom=fulltext
- http://www.jbc.org/content/293/15/5425.abstract
- http://www.clinsci.org/image-gallery/autophagy
- http://www.tmd.ac.jp/english/artis-cms/cms-files/Autophagy.pdf
- http://mcr.aacrjournals.org/content/early/2018/05/19/1541-7786.MCR-17-0634
- http://square.umin.ac.jp/molbiol/english/index.html
- http://cib.csic.es/research/cellular-and-molecular-biology/roles-autophagy-health-and-disease
- https://www.nytimes.com/2016/10/04/science/yoshinori-ohsumi-nobel-prize-medicine.html
- https://www.invivogen.com/autophagy
- http://www.med.monash.edu.au/biochem/labs/lazarou-lab.html
- https://journals.lww.com/co-criticalcare/Abstract/2018/04000/Autophagy___should_it_play_a_role_in_ICU.9.aspx

36353751R00060

Printed in Great Britain
by Amazon